D1290983

To our long-suffering families at home, namely, husband George and sons Benjamin and Christopher at the Lifeboat station on Glasgow Green; and the lovely Emma and beautiful daughters Kate, Charlotte and Maisie in sunny Bearsden.

Problem Solving in
Infection

Edited by

STEPHANIE J. DANCER, BSc, MB BS, MSc, MD, FRCPath, DTM&H
Consultant Microbiologist, NHS Lanarkshire, Scotland

R. ANDREW SEATON, MBChB, MD, DTM&H, FRCP (Edinburgh & Glasgow)
Consultant in Infectious Diseases and General Medicine, Honorary Senior Lecturer,
University of Glasgow, Brownlee Centre for Infectious Diseases and Tropical Medicine,
Gartnavel General Hospital, Glasgow, UK

CLINICAL PUBLISHING
OXFORD

CLINICAL PUBLISHING
an imprint of Atlas Medical Publishing Ltd

Oxford Centre for Innovation
Mill Street, Oxford OX2 0JX, UK

Tel: +44 1865 811116
Fax: +44 1865 251550
E mail: info@clinicalpublishing.co.uk
Web: www.clinicalpublishing.co.uk

Distributed in USA and Canada by:
Clinical Publishing
30 Amberwood Parkway
Ashland OH 44805 USA
tel: 800-247-6553 (toll free within US and Canada)
fax: 419-281-6883
email: order@bookmasters.com

Distributed in UK and Rest of World by:
Marston Book Services Ltd
PO Box 269
Abingdon
Oxon OX14 4YN UK
tel: +44 1235 465500
fax: +44 1235 465555
email: trade.orders@marston.co.uk

A catalogue record for this book is available from the British Library.

ISBN 13   978 1 904392 83 5
ISBN e-book 978 1 84692 625 9

Project manager: Gavin Smith, GPS Publishing Solutions, Herts, UK
Typeset by Phoenix Photosetting, Chatham, UK

Printed by Marston Book Services Ltd, Abingdon, Oxon., UK

Contents

SECTION 3   Infections in Special Circumstances

Infections in Critical Care

Immunocompromised Patient

Preface

This collection of clinical cases has been written by specialists and practitioners in infectious diseases, clinical microbiology and others with an interest in infection within their own speciality. Contributors are based at UK hospitals and further afield. The material is aimed at medical students, microbiology and infectious diseases trainees and generalist clinicians. We hope it will also be useful to other medical and non-medical professionals working, training or just interested in infection-related specialties. The cases draw on real-life clinical situations within adult hospital practice. Whilst the majority of cases relate to commonly encountered or less common but serious infections, we have also included rarer or emerging infections, particularly when they illustrate broader principles of infection management and prevention. We hope these cases will help bring the reader up to date in some of the key areas relating to contemporary diagnosis and management of infection in the setting of a developed healthcare system. Most importantly, we hope the reader will be informed, entertained and stimulated to read more about the fascinating subject of infectious diseases. We would like to take the opportunity to thank all our friends and colleagues at home and abroad who have made this book possible, including a special thank-you to Jane Pennington, who should take full responsibility for its genesis.

SJD
RAS
November, 2011

Contributors

Dugal Baird, Retired Consultant Medical Microbiologist, Hairmyres Hospital, NHS Lanarkshire, East Kilbride, UK

Gavin Barlow, Consultant in Infectious Diseases, Castle Hill Hospital, Hull and East Yorkshire Hospitals NHS Trust, Hull, UK

Stephen Barrett, Consultant Medical Microbiologist, Southend Hospital NHS Trust, Southend, Essex, UK

Vhairi M. Bateman, Specialist Registrar in Infectious Diseases and Microbiology, Aberdeen Royal Infirmary, NHS Grampian, Aberdeen, UK

Sophie Beal, Former Specialist Registrar in Obstetrics and Gynaecology, St James' Hospital, Leeds, UK

Andrew Berrington, Consultant Medical Microbiologist, Sunderland Royal Hospital, City Hospitals Sunderland NHS Foundation Trust, Sunderland, UK

Alec Bonington, Consultant in Infectious Diseases, North Manchester General Hospital, Penine Acute Hospitals NHS Trust, Manchester, UK

Adam Bowman, Consultant in Elderly Care Medicine, Glasgow Royal Infirmary, NHS Greater Glasgow and Clyde, Glasgow, UK

Stewart Campbell, Consultant Gastroenterologist, Hairmyres Hospital, NHS Lanarkshire, East Kilbride, UK

Paul Chadwick, Consultant Microbiologist, Salford Hospital, Salford Royal NHS Trust, Salford, UK

Ann Chapman, Consultant in Infectious Diseases, Royal Hallamshire Hospital, Sheffield Teaching Hospitals NHS Trust, Sheffield, UK

Bart J. Currie, Professor of Tropical and Emerging Infectious Diseases, Menzies School of Health Research, Darwin, Australia

Stephanie J. Dancer, Consultant Medical Microbiologist, Hairmyres Hospital, NHS Lanarkshire, East Kilbride, UK

Christopher Duncan, Research Fellow, Sir William Dunn School of Pathology, University of Oxford, Oxford, UK

Stephanie Dundas, Consultant in Infectious Diseases and General Medicine, Monklands General Hospital, NHS Lanarkshire, Airdrie, UK

Dale Fisher, Associate Professor and Specialist in Infectious Diseases, National University Hospital, Singapore

Vance Fowler, Associate Professor and Infectious Diseases Specialist, Department of Medicine, Duke University Medical Center, Durham, North Carolina, USA

Alan P. Gibb, Consultant Medical Microbiologist, Royal Infirmary of Edinburgh, NHS Lothian Health Board, Edinburgh, UK

Iain Gould, Consultant Medical Microbiologist, Aberdeen Royal Infirmary, NHS Grampian, Aberdeen, UK

Achyut Guleri, Consultant Medical Microbiologist, Blackpool Victoria Hospital, Blackpool, Fylde and Wyre Hospitals NHS Foundation Trust, UK

Emma Louise Hathorn, Specialist Registrar in Genitourinary Medicine, Whittall Street Clinic, Heart of Birmingham Teaching NHS Primary Care Trust, Birmingham, UK

Carolyn Hemsley, Consultant in Infectious Diseases and Medical Microbiology, St Thomas' Hospital, Guy's and St Thomas' NHS Foundation Trust, London, UK

Antonia Ho, Specialist Registrar in Infectious Diseases, Gartnavel General Hospital, NHS Greater Glasgow and Clyde, Glasgow, UK

Dermot Kennedy, Retired Consultant in Infectious Diseases, Gartnavel General Hospital, NHS Greater Glasgow and Clyde, Glasgow, UK

Nicholas Kennedy, Consultant in Infectious Diseases and General Medicine, Monklands General Hospital, NHS Lanarkshire, Airdrie, UK

Kevin Kerr, Professor and Consultant Medical Microbiologist, Harrogate General Hospital, Harrogate and District NHS Foundation Trust, Harrogate, UK

Alisdair A. MacConnachie, Consultant in Infectious diseases, Gartnavel General Hospital, NHS Greater Glasgow and Clyde, Glasgow, UK

Alexander Mackenzie, Consultant in Infectious Diseases and General Medicine, Aberdeen Royal Infirmary, NHS Grampian Health Board, Aberdeen, UK

Claire Mackintosh, Consultant in Infectious Diseases, Western General Hospital, NHS Lothian Health Board, Edinburgh, UK

Marina Morgan, Consultant Medical Microbiologist, Royal Devon and Exeter Hospital, Royal Devon and Exeter NHS Foundation Trust, Exeter, UK

Nneka Nwokolo, Consultant in Genitourinary Medicine, Chelsea and Westminster Hospital, Chelsea and Westminster NHS Foundation Trust, London, UK

Beryl Oppenheim, Consultant Microbiologist, City Hospital, Sandwell and West Birmingham Hospitals NHS Trust, Birmingham, UK

Thomas Patterson, Professor of Medicine and Infectious Diseases, University of Texas Health Science Center, San Antonio, Texas, USA

Lynette Pereira, Yong Loo Lin School of Medicine, National University Singapore, Singapore

Christine Peters, Specialist Registrar in Medical Microbiology, Southern General Hospital, NHS Greater Glasgow and Clyde, Glasgow, UK

Erica Peters, Consultant in Infectious Diseases, Gartnavel General Hospital, NHS Greater Glasgow and Clyde, Glasgow, UK

Christopher D. Pfeiffer, Clinical Fellow, Department of Medicine, Duke University Medical Center, Durham, North Carolina, USA

Michael Przybylo, Registrar in Medical Microbiology, Blackpool Victoria Hospital, Blackpool, Fylde and Wyre Hospitals NHS Foundation Trust, UK

Neil D. Ritchie, Clinical Lecturer in Infectious Diseases, Medical Faculty, University of Glasgow, Glasgow, UK

Paul Robertson, Associate Specialist in Clinical Microbiology and Infectious Diseases, Monklands General Hospital, NHS Lanarkshire, Airdrie, UK

Kevin Rooney, Consultant in Intensive Care Medicine and Professor of Care Improvement, School of Health, Nursing and Midwifery, University of the West of Scotland, Paisley, UK

R. Andrew Seaton, Consultant in Infectious Diseases, Gartnavel General Hospital, NHS Greater Glasgow and Clyde, Glasgow, UK

Rashmi Sharma, Consultant Medical Microbiologist, Blackpool Victoria Hospital, Blackpool, Fylde and Wyre Hospitals NHS Foundation Trust, UK

Lee Stewart, Antimicrobial Pharmacist, Southern General Hospital, NHS Greater Glasgow and Clyde, Glasgow, UK

Alison H. Thomson, Senior Lecturer in Clinical Pharmacy, Department of Pharmacy, University of Strathclyde, Glasgow, UK

Andrew J. Winter, Consultant in Genitourinary Medicine, Sandyford Centre, NHS Greater Glasgow and Clyde, Glasgow, UK

Beth White, Specialist Registrar in Infectious Diseases, Gartnavel General Hospital, NHS Greater Glasgow and Clyde, Glasgow

Helena White, Specialist Registrar in Infectious Diseases, Leicester Royal Infirmary, University of Leicester Hospitals NHS Trust, Leicester, UK

Sarah Whitehead, Consultant in Medical Microbiology, Southern General Hospital, NHS Greater Glasgow and Clyde, Glasgow, UK

Abbreviations

3GC	third-generation cephalosporins	EEG	electroencephalography
AFFB	acid-fast bacilli stain	eGFR	estimated glomerular filtration rate
AIDS	acquired immune deficiency syndrome	EIA	enzyme immunoassay
APRV	airway pressure release ventilation	ELISA	enzyme-linked immunosorbent assay
ARDS	acute respiratory distress syndrome	ENT	ear, nose and throat
ART	antiretroviral therapy	ESBL	extended spectrum β-lactamase
AXR	abdominal X-ray	FiO$_2$	inspired oxygen concentration
AZT	zidovudine	G6PD	glucose 6-phosphate dehydrogenase
BAL	bronchoalveolar lavage		
BHIVA	British HIV Association	GAS	Group A beta-haemolytic *Streptococcus*
BM	bacterial meningitis		
BNF	British National Formulary	GBS	group B *Streptococcus*
BP	blood pressure	GCS	Glasgow Coma Scale
CA-MRSA	community-acquired methicillin-resistant *Staphylococcus aureus*	GI	gastrointestinal
		GMP	good manufacturing practice
CAP	community-acquired pneumonia	GP	general practitioner
CDAD	*Clostridium difficile*-associated diarrhoea	HAART	highly active antiretroviral therapy
		HAI	healthcare-associated infection
CDC	Centers for Disease Control and Prevention	HA-MRSA	healthcare-associated methicillin-resistant *Staphylococcus aureus*
CDI	*Clostridium difficile* infection	HAV	hepatitis A virus
CHB	chronic hepatitis B	HBsAg	hepatitis B surface antigen
CMV	cytomegalovirus	HBV	hepatitis B virus
CNS	coagulase-negative staphylococci	HCV	hepatitis C virus
COPD	chronic obstructive pulmonary disease	HDV	hepatitis Delta virus
		Hep B	hepatitis B
CPIS	Clinical Pulmonary Infection Score	Hep C	hepatitis C
CRP	C-reactive protein	HFOV	high-frequency oscillatory ventilation
CSF	cerebrospinal fluid		
CT	computed tomography	HIV	human immunodeficiency virus
CXR	chest X-ray	HSE	herpes simplex encephalitis
DDD	defined daily dose	HSV	herpes simplex virus
DF2	Dysgonic Fermenter type 2	HUS	haemolytic uraemic syndrome
DFI	diabetic foot infections	I&D	incision and drainage
DIC	disseminated intravascular coagulation	IAP	intravenous antibiotic prophylaxis
		ICN	infection control nurse
DOT	directly observed therapy	ICP	intracranial pressure
EBV	Epstein–Barr virus	ICU	intensive care unit
ECMO	extracorporeal membrane oxygenation	IDU	injecting drug use
		IDUs	injecting drug users

IE	infective endocarditis	pO$_2$	oxygen pressure
IgG	immunoglobulin G	PPROM	pre-term premature rupture of
IgM	immunoglobulin M		membranes
IJV	internal jugular vein	PVL	Panton-Valentine leukocidin
IL-6	interleukin-6	RBC	red blood cell
ILI	influenza-like illness	rBPI	recombinant bactericidal/
IRIS	immune reconstitution		permeability-increasing protein
	inflammatory syndrome	RCOG	Royal College of Obstetricians and
ITU	Intensive Therapy Unit		Gynaecologists
IV	intravenous	RCT	randomized controlled trial
IVIG	intravenous immunoglobulin G	RDT	rapid diagnostic test
LD	Legionnaires' disease	RT-PCR	reverse transcriptase–polymerase
LDH	lactate dehydrogenase		chain reaction
LGV	lymphogranuloma venereum	SARS	severe acute respiratory syndrome
LOC	level of consciousness	SBP	spontaneous bacterial peritonitis
LP	lumbar puncture	SDD	selective digestive tract
MAOI	monoamine oxidase inhibitor		decontamination
MDRTB	multidrug-resistant tuberculosis	SIRS	systemic inflammatory response
MHC	major histocompatibility complex		syndrome
MIC	minimum inhibitory	SpO$_2$	saturation of peripheral oxygen
	concentration	SSC	Surviving Sepsis Campaign
MRI	magnetic resonance imaging	SSTI	skin and soft tissue infection
MRSA	methicillin-resistant *Staphylococcus*	STEC	Shiga toxin-producing *Escherichia*
	aureus		*coli*
MSM	men who have sex with men	STI	sexually transmitted infection
MSQ	mental state questionnaire	STSS	streptococcal toxic shock
MSSA	methicillin-susceptible		syndrome
	Staphylococcus aureus	TB	tuberculosis
MSSU	mid-stream specimen of urine	TNF-α	tumour necrosis factor alpha
NAAT	nucleic acid amplification test	TOE	trans-oesophageal echocardiogram
NF	necrotizing fasciitis	TPPA	*Treponema pallidum* particle
NICE	National Institute for Health and		agglutination
	Clinical Excellence	TSS	toxic shock syndrome
NMB	neuromuscular blocking agent	TTE	trans-thoracic echocardiogram
NSTI	necrotizing soft tissue infection	URTI	upper respiratory tract infection
OHPAT	outpatient and home parenteral	UTI	urinary tract infection
	antimicrobial therapy	VAP	ventilator-associated pneumonia
OI	opportunistic infections	VDRL	venereal disease research
PaO$_2$	partial pressure of arterial oxygen		laboratory
PCIRV	pressure control inverse ratio	VP	ventriculoperitoneal
	ventilation	VRE	vancomycin-resistant enterococci
PCP	*Pneumocystis jirovecii* pneumonia	VT	tidal volume
PCR	polymerase chain reaction	VTEC	verocytotoxin-producing
PEG-INF	pegylated interferon		*Escherichia coli*
PEP	post-exposure prophylaxis	WCC	white blood cell count
PHI	primary HIV infection	WHO	World Health Organization
PJI	prosthetic joint infection	XDRTB	extensively drug-resistant
			tuberculosis

Principles

THE PATIENT WITH SEPSIS

PROBLEM

1   Assessment of the Patient with Sepsis

R. Andrew Seaton

Case History

A previously healthy 19-year-old woman presented to her general practitioner with fever, myalgia, sore throat and fatigue. Her temperature was 38.2°C, heart rate 100 beats/min and respiratory rate 22 breaths/min. The pharynx was inflamed with moderate exudate. Blood pressure was 100/60 mmHg. She looked well and viral upper respiratory tract infection was suspected. A throat swab for bacteria and viruses was performed and analgesics prescribed. Twelve hours later she collapsed and was taken to the emergency department. A widespread macular rash was evident on the trunk (Figure 1.1), heart rate was 130 beats/min, respiratory rate 34 breaths/min, blood pressure 70/40 mmHg and temperature 39°C. *Streptococcus pyogenes* was isolated from the throat swab.

What are the key clinical indicators of infection and its severity?

What is the likely cause of this person's collapse?

How should this patient be managed?

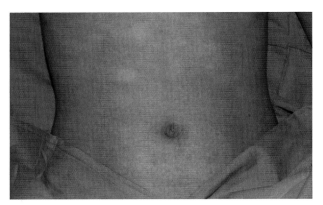

Figure 1.1 A widespread macular rash on the trunk (*see inside front cover for colour version*).

Background

The systemic inflammatory response syndrome (SIRS) reflects the host immune response, including the release of pro-inflammatory cytokines, to a variety of stimuli (infection, ischaemia, chemical toxins, vasculitis and trauma). SIRS is defined by at least two key clinical (fever, hypothermia, tachycardia and tachypnoea) or laboratory (neutrophil leukocytosis or leukopenia) signs of inflammation (Table 1.1). Clinical symptoms and signs of infection in conjunction with SIRS define 'sepsis'. Severe sepsis is sepsis with associated organ dysfunction, hypoperfusion or hypotension. Originally proposed to give consistency in patient assessment for clinical trials in severe infection, these criteria have been shown to correlate well with outcome in everyday clinical practice with mortality increasing with sepsis severity. Septic shock has the poorest prognosis with mortality >50%. In general, sepsis syndrome is a manifestation of serious bacterial infection but it may also be a manifestation of other infections including viraemia (e.g. influenza, measles), parasitaemia (e.g. falciparum malaria) and fungaemia (e.g. candidaemia). Bacterial sepsis is associated with bacteraemia and may be triggered by a number of mechanisms including release of endotoxin (e.g. in Gram-negative infection) or exotoxin release as is seen in staphylococcal or streptococcal toxic shock syndrome (TSS). Early recognition of SIRS, sepsis and severe sepsis should institute prompt targeted antimicrobial therapy against the most likely organisms. Choice of agent will be guided by the anatomical and systemic manifestations of infection and associated epidemiological risk factors (Table 1.2). In true community-acquired sepsis in the UK, the most commonly isolated organisms from blood cultures are *Escherichia coli* (urinary tract source), *Streptococcus pneumoniae* (pneumonia) and *Staphylococcus aureus* (soft tissue or primary bacteraemia). *Streptococcus pyogenes* (Group A beta-haemolytic *Streptococcus* [GAS]) and *Neisseria meningitidis* are important additional risks particularly in younger adults and children.

Toxic shock syndrome

TSS is a severe and life-threatening condition caused typically by either GAS or methicillin-sensitive or methicillin-resistant *Staphylococcus aureus*. TSS has also been described

Table 1.1 Symptoms and signs of the systemic inflammatory response syndrome (SIRS)

SIRS if ≥2 of:		SEPSIS	Severe SEPSIS = SEPSIS + one of:
Tachycardia	Heart rate >90 beats/min	SIRS + symptoms/signs of infection (e.g. rigors, dysuria, erythema, purulent sputum, presence of pus, etc.)	Hypotension: systolic blood pressure ≤90 mmHg despite fluid resuscitation or vasopressor/inotropic support required
Tachypnoea	Respiratory rate >20 breaths/min		Adult respiratory distress syndrome: acute onset of diffuse pulmonary infiltrates and hypoxaemia in the absence of cardiac failure or by evidence of diffuse capillary leak manifested by acute onset of generalized or pleural oedema
Fever or hypothermia	Temperature <36°C or >38°C		Acidosis (blood lactate >4 mmol/l)
			Coagulopathy (disseminated intravascular coagulation or thrombocytopenia, platelet count <100 × 10^9/l)
Leukocytosis or leukopenia	Peripheral white blood cell count <4 or >12 × 10^9/l or band forms present on blood film		Renal failure: oliguria or rising creatinine
			Hepatic dysfunction: increasing bilirubin or transaminases
			Acute alteration in mental status

Table 1.2 Examples of epidemiological risk factors for infection

Risk factor	Nature of risk/infection type	Notable organisms
Healthcare–associated infection (including recent hospitalization or surgery)	Vascular device, urinary catheter related, metalwork/surgery associated, ventilator associated or antibiotic therapy induced. Bloodstream, urinary tract, respiratory tract and enteric infections	*Staphylococcus aureus* (including MRSA), coagulase-negative staphylococci, enterococci, *Clostridium difficile*, resistant Gram-negative infection (e.g. extended spectrum β-lactamase-producing organisms)
Immunosuppressive states and agents	Multiple risks including chemotherapy, biological agents, other rheumatic disease-modifying agents, transplantation antirejection therapy, corticosteroids, malignancy, advanced HIV	Additional risk of opportunistic organisms including low-virulence bacteria, fungi (*Candida, Aspergillus*) and viruses (cytomegalovirus)
Diabetes	Risk factors include vascular disease, impaired humoral immunity, neuropathy. Soft tissue, osteomyelitis, pneumonia, urinary tract	*S. aureus*, streptococci, pneumococci, fungi (*Candida, Aspergillus*)
Parenteral drug misuse	Soft tissue infection, vascular infection, endocarditis, pneumonia, blood-borne virus	*S. aureus*, streptococci, clostridial species, pneumococci
Alcohol excess and chronic liver disease	Pneumonia, spontaneous bacterial peritonitis, meningitis	Pneumococci, listeriosis, streptococci, Gram-negative infection
Occupation and environment	Environmental and zoonotic risk	Leptospirosis, *E. coli* O157, *Coxiella burnetii*
Travel	Nature/region of travel/activities, travel itinerary, rural versus urban, immunization and prophylaxis history	Malaria, enteric fever, Dengue, Rickettsia, meningococci, leptospirosis, imported resistant bacteria (e.g. penicillin-resistant pneumococci

HIV, human immunodeficiency virus; MRSA, methicillin-resistant *Staphylococcus aureus* with other beta-haemolytic streptococci. In both GAS and *S. aureus* TSS, pyrogenic exotoxins or superantigens are produced which interact directly with the host class II major histocompatibility complex (MHC) molecules. These bind to T-cell receptors and trigger massive polyclonal T-cell activation and a resultant cytokine storm including tumour necrosis factor alpha (TNF-α) and interleukin-6 (IL-6). In GAS TSS, the streptococcal M protein within the cell wall binds to host complement regulators and impedes phagocytosis by mononuclear cells. Clinically, GAS and *S. aureus* TSS may be difficult to differentiate as both are characterized by hypotension and erythroderma. GAS TSS is associated with higher mortality (up to 80%) and there should be clinical and microbiological evidence of GAS, usually a necrotizing soft tissue infection or pharyngitis. Strict definition of GAS TSS requires the presence of hypotension and at least two other features of multiorgan dysfunction (Table 1.3). Lack of multiorgan involvement and hypotension differentiates 'scarlet fever' from GAS TSS. Staphylococcal TSS is less common and has an attributable mortality of about 5%. It typically occurs in young women and is associated with tampon use, menses and intravaginal contraceptive devices but may also complicate skin infections, particularly after surgical procedures. Microbiological tests are typically negative. The diagnosis of staphylococcal TSS is confirmed in the presence of fever, macular rash (which desquamates 1–2 weeks after onset), hypotension and evidence of multiorgan involvement and no positive microbiological cultures (excepting *S. aureus*) (Table 1.3). In the illustrative case, isolation of GAS from the throat swab differentiates between streptococcal and staphylococcal TSS.

Table 1.3 Clinical features of GAS and *S. aureus* TSS

	GAS TSS	*S. aureus* TSS
Hypotension	Always	Always
Fever	Usual	Always
Generalized erythroderma	Usual	Always
Desquamation	May occur	Usual 1–2 weeks after onset
Soft tissue infection	If soft tissue primary site: necrotizing fasciitis, myositis or gangrene	Infrequently primary site. May occur post-operatively
Case definition	Hypotension, microbiological evidence of GAS infection and ≥2 of: rash, soft tissue necrosis, renal dysfunction, coagulopathy (thrombocytopenia or disseminated intravascular coagulation), hepatic dysfunction, ARDS, new-onset confusion	Fever, rash (with desquamation) and hypotension. Other pathogens excluded although *S. aureus* may be isolated and ≥3 of: vomiting/diarrhoea at onset, severe myalgia or creatinine phosphokinase twice normal, mucous membrane hyperaemia, renal dysfunction, thrombocytopenia, hepatic dysfunction, central nervous system involvement

ARDS, acute respiratory distress syndrome

Management of sepsis and TSS

In the septic patient, blood culture is mandatory as is rapid identification and removal of any potential source of infection (e.g. infected vascular catheter or abscess collection). Empirical parenteral antimicrobial therapy should be administered promptly after blood cultures. Notably in severe streptococcal infections, where there is a large bacterial load, a high rate of treatment failure with penicillin has been observed. In animal models, clindamycin use has been associated with considerably greater success than penicillin, particularly when therapy is delayed. In these circumstances a stationary growth phase of GAS is reached quickly and *in vitro* experiments have demonstrated that critical penicillin-binding proteins are not expressed at this time, so potentially rendering β-lactam antibiotics ineffective. In contrast to β-lactams, clindamycin maintains activity against GAS irrespective of the growth phase. It is also a potent suppressor of bacterial toxin synthesis and may facilitate phagocytosis of *S. pyogenes* by inhibiting M protein synthesis.

Early physiological supportive measures, in addition to antibiotic management, are extremely important in sepsis including TSS. Severe sepsis should be managed in a high-dependency or intensive care setting. Supportive measures include intravascular volume resuscitation with crystalloid or colloid to improve filling pressure ('goal-directed therapy'), optimization of oxygenation and ventilation (due to the associated ventilation–perfusion abnormalities), correction of acidosis and renal and inotrope/vasopressor support. Adjunctive measures which have been shown to be of benefit in subsets of patients with severe sepsis in the intensive care setting include stress-dose corticosteroids (in adults with septic shock only after blood pressure has been shown to be poorly responsive to fluid and vasopressor therapy) and recombinant activated protein C (in adult patients judged to be at high risk for death by the presence of multiorgan failure and without contraindications based on bleeding risk).

Recent Developments

Despite prompt antibiotic therapy, mortality in GAS TSS remains high and there is a need for specific adjuvant therapy. Lack of protective humoral immunity against GAS virulence factors is thought to contribute to susceptibility to invasive infection and so adjunctive human polyspecific intravenous immunoglobulin G (IVIG) therapy has been proposed. IVIG is able to neutralize a wide variety of superantigens and to facilitate opsonization of GAS. To date the only placebo-controlled randomized trial of IVIG in GAS TSS was terminated prematurely because of slow patient recruitment. Although only 21 patients were enrolled in this multicentre study, there was a 3.6-fold increase in mortality in placebo recipients and a significant increase in plasma neutralizing activity against superantigens expressed by autologous isolates in IVIG-treated patients. Although administration of IVIG therapy for GAS TSS is now widely practised, larger studies are required to corroborate these findings and to better guide clinicians in IVIG use.

Conclusion

Significant improvements have been achieved in the support of patients with severe sepsis in recent years; however, mortality remains high. It therefore remains critical that early signs of sepsis are recognized quickly both in the community and hospital and that appropriate investigations and management are initiated rapidly before severe sepsis ensues.

Further Reading

Bone RC, Balk RA, Cerra FB *et al*. Definitions for sepsis and organ failure and guidelines for the use of innovative therapies in sepsis. *Chest* 1992; **101**: 1644–55.

Darenberg J, Ihendyane N, Sjölin J *et al*. Intravenous immunoglobulin G therapy in streptococcal toxic shock syndrome: a European randomized, double-blind, placebo-controlled trial. *Clin Infect Dis* 2003; **37**: 333–40.

Dellinger RP, Levy MM, Carlet JM *et al*. Surviving Sepsis Campaign: international guidelines for management of severe sepsis and septic shock: 2008. *Crit Care Med* 2008; **36**: 296–327.

Lesher L, DeVries A, Danila R, Lynfield R. Evaluation of surveillance methods for staphylococcal toxic shock syndrome. *Emerg Infect Dis* 2009; **15**: 770–3.

Stevens DL. The flesh-eating bacterium: what's next? *J Infect Dis* 1999: **179**(Suppl 2): S366–74.

PROBLEM

2 Assessing Sepsis in the Elderly

Adam Bowman

Case History

A 78-year-old man resident in a nursing home presented to the emergency department. He had previously had a stroke and had a long-term urethral catheter *in situ*. He had been unwell for several days and on initial assessment was confused and drowsy with a blood pressure of 90/40 mmHg and temperature of 37.5°C. His dipstick urinalysis was positive for blood, leukocytes and nitrites. Intravenous co-amoxiclav was started for a presumed urinary tract infection and he initially improved. Several days later, however, he became unwell again, with fever and profuse diarrhoea.

What clinical features are there in this man's initial presentation to suggest an underlying diagnosis of sepsis?

Was his initial antibiotic therapy appropriate and are there any special considerations that should guide empirical antimicrobial prescribing in patients such as this?

Background

Sepsis is a major cause of morbidity and mortality in the elderly population and mortality due to sepsis increases in a linear manner with age. Sepsis is a leading cause of hospitalization in this age group. Common sites of infection in elderly patients include the respiratory tract (50% of all cases of pneumonia occur in patients over 65 years of age), urinary tract, and skin and soft tissues. The initial approach to investigation and management of the older patient with sepsis is in essence the same as that for any patient presenting with presumed sepsis. There are, however, important subtleties and pitfalls to be aware of when dealing with sepsis in this patient population.

In elderly patients, multiple predisposing factors provide increased exposure to pathogens and allow infection and subsequent sepsis to develop. Extrinsic factors include comorbidity, poor functional status, immobility, institutionalization, repeated invasive procedures (such as catheterization) and recurrent hospital admissions. Intrinsic factors include age-related changes in immune function, altered homeostasis and decreased cardiopulmonary reserve.

All of the factors noted above have been identified as contributors to the development of sepsis in the elderly; it is readily apparent that many of these apply to the very typical patient outlined above.

It has long been recognized that sepsis may present atypically in elderly patients and this can pose a significant diagnostic challenge to clinicians. Changes in immune function with increasing age (immunosenescence) and altered homeostatic mechanisms mean that the typical presenting features of sepsis may not be present in older patients. Fever response, for example, often the cardinal presenting sign suggesting sepsis, may be blunted or absent, and a significant proportion of elderly patients with bacteraemia will never exhibit a significant fever. It follows therefore that absence of fever cannot rule out infection in these patients. The clinical presentation of sepsis in elderly patients may be very non-specific with weakness, general malaise and falls being common presenting features. Delirium (acute confusional state) is an extremely common presenting feature of sepsis in older adults, particularly in those with multiple comorbidities or pre-existing cognitive impairment. It is important to determine if the confusion is of new onset or worsening of a long-standing confusional state. In this regard, confirmatory history from a carer is essential. Any acute change in cognition or change in functional status in an elderly patient should alert the clinician to the possibility of underlying infection and initial investigations should reflect this.

Initial assessment and management

Regardless of age, initial investigation of the patient presenting with sepsis should be directed towards confirming the diagnosis of infection (routine blood tests, blood cultures, urine cultures, etc.), assessing for possible sources of infection (clinical examination, chest X-ray, etc.) and assessing the severity of sepsis. Urinary catheters (as in this case) are frequently colonized with bacteria, making assessment of urinalysis and culture difficult.

The initial management of sepsis in the elderly should follow the guidelines outlined by the Surviving Sepsis Campaign, with the emphasis (as in any septic patient) on maintaining perfusion pressure via fluid resuscitation ± inotropic support, source identification and early administration of appropriate empirical antibiotic therapy. Removal or replacement of medical devices which may be a potential source of infection, such as intravascular or (as in this case) urinary catheters, should be considered in all patients with sepsis and is mandatory if the source of sepsis is not known.

Initial empirical antibiotic choices are similar in all patients regardless of age, with a few important additional points to consider in older patients. In patients with significant comorbidity, repeated antimicrobial exposure and recurrent hospitalization are common and therefore levels of antimicrobial resistance may be higher. Changes in pharmacokinetics with increasing age may make antibiotic dosing more difficult and older patients are at higher risk of developing side effects and complications related to antimicrobial use. Frail elderly patients are at a particularly high risk of developing *Clostridium difficile* infection which is frequently associated with poor outcome in this patient group. This is due to a combination of increased prevalence of risk factors which predispose to *C. difficile* infection (comorbidities, recurrent hospital admission, use of agents to suppress gastric acid, etc.) and the presence of factors known to be associated with poor outcomes (hypoalbuminaemia, renal failure, functional impairment, etc.), all of which are more common in frail elderly people. Empirical antimicrobial regimens for these patients should take all of the above into account, as well as likely pathogen and source of infection, and agents less likely to encourage *C. difficile* should be used. Initial antibiotic cover should be rationalized to targeted therapy as soon as culture results allow, and antibiotic regimens limiting the use of antibiotics associated with increased risk of healthcare-associated infections (quinolones, cephalosporins, co-amoxiclav, etc.) should be considered.

Further Considerations

In the case above, where urinary sepsis was suspected, the urinary catheter should be removed and replaced. Although intravenous co-amoxiclav successfully treated this man's urinary sepsis, its use may well have contributed to the subsequent development of *C. difficile*-associated diarrhoea. It would have been preferable in this case to have used an age-, weight- and creatinine-adjusted intravenous dose of gentamicin as empirical cover pending blood and urine culture results. Gentamicin-induced renal, oto- and vestibular toxicity in the elderly is well recognized but can be minimized with short-duration therapy (72 hours or less) and by careful monitoring of blood concentrations and renal function. A switch to an appropriate oral agent may be possible at that stage. Other agents useful in lower urinary tract infection and less likely to encourage *C. difficile* include nitrofurantoin, trimethoprim and co-trimoxazole. Oral options for upper urinary tract infections with lower propensity for *C. difficile* infection are more limited but include co-trimoxazole and amoxicillin following isolation of a susceptible organism.

While many elderly patients presenting with sepsis will respond well to the management strategies outlined above, it is worth remembering that an episode of severe sepsis/septic shock will be a terminal event for a proportion of elderly patients. In these cases appropriate management will involve end-of-life care, which may in turn involve decisions regarding withholding or withdrawal of treatment. Such decisions invariably raise a number of ethical issues and should always be made by senior members of the medical team, taking cognisance of the patient's pre-expressed wishes.

Conclusion

- Sepsis is common in elderly patients.
- The clinical presentation may be atypical leading to difficulty in making the diagnosis.

- Delirium is an extremely common presenting feature and its presence should always prompt a search for underlying infection.
- The principles of initial assessment and management of sepsis are the same in all patients regardless of age.

Further Reading

Dellinger RP, Carlet JM, Masur H *et al*. Surviving Sepsis Campaign guidelines for management of severe sepsis and septic shock. *Crit Care Med* 2004; **32**: 858–73.

Girard TD, Opal SM, Ely EW. Insights into severe sepsis in older patients: from epidemiology to evidence-based management. *Clin Infect Dis* 2005; **40**: 719–27.

Martin GS, Mannino DM, Moss M. The effect of age on the development and outcome of adult sepsis. *Crit Care Med* 2006; **34**: 15–21.

Moran D. Infections in the elderly. *Top Emerg Med* 2003; **25**: 174–81.

PROBLEM

3 Updating Infection Prevention and Control

Stephanie J. Dancer

Case History

Dr Barry is a senior physician in a district general hospital. He has been asked to review the delivery of infection control in the hospital following a request from the hospital's Board of Directors. He has no previous experience other than awareness of screening activities for methicillin-resistant *Staphylococcus aureus* (MRSA). There is one infection control nurse (ICN) assisted by a part-time staff nurse on secondment. There is also an on-site microbiology laboratory but the microbiologist is off on long-term sick leave with cover obtained from another healthcare Trust. How should Dr Barry proceed? The year before, there was an extensive outbreak of norovirus affecting the whole hospital, and rates of MRSA and *Clostridium difficile* infection have recently escalated on the long-term care wards.

What is the first thing that Dr Barry should do?

What are the most important issues to tackle?

What longer-term plans could be initiated?

Background

Healthcare-associated infection (HAI) occurs when a patient acquires an infection in a healthcare establishment that was neither present nor incubating on admission. HAI is costly, inconvenient and dangerous. There is therefore an obligation for hospitals to put into place policies, procedures and guidelines in order to reduce the risk of HAI for patients as far as possible. These are the principles underpinning infection control, and the responsibility for its structure and efficiency should not be underestimated.

The most common hospital pathogens include MRSA, *C. difficile*, multidrug-resistant Gram-negative bacilli, vancomycin-resistant enterococci (VRE) and norovirus. Such organisms thrive in the close confines of the hospital environment, subject to antibiotic pressures and a variety of infection control interventions. Protecting the patient from infection requires multifaceted activity at all levels involving clinical and non-clinical staff, managers, visitors and patients themselves. Given the number of different staff who could potentially contribute towards a review of HAI strategies, the first action is to organize a short-life infection control group for the hospital.

Box 3.1 lists key staff invited to the infection control review group.

Box 3.1 Members of the infection control review group.

- Senior physician (chairman)
- Infection control nurse and staff nurse (ICNs)
- Consultant microbiologist or representative
- Senior hospital manager and/or member of Board of Directors
- Pharmacist
- Consultant or deputy representing care of the elderly
- Consultant intensivist or deputy representing intensive care unit
- Occupational health doctor
- Clinical director in surgery
- Senior nurse manager
- Estates manager
- Domestic services supervisor
- Catering manager
- Theatre sister
- Patient representative
- Consultant in public health medicine or deputy
- Secretary

Infection control review: inaugural meeting

Since the medical microbiologist was absent, a biomedical scientist represented the microbiology laboratory at the meeting. There were a number of items on the HAI agenda to discuss but the first item to receive attention was hand hygiene (Box 3.2).

Hand hygiene compliance

Despite regular overt surveillance, compliance was generally poor and it was agreed to launch a campaign to raise awareness. This would include notices and visual alerts

---

Box 3.2 Agenda for inaugural meeting of the infection control review group.

1. Apologies
2. Welcome and introduction of staff
3. Confidentiality disclosures and conflicts of interest
4. Infection control objectives and current status
5. Areas of responsibility
6. Matters arising: hand hygiene; antimicrobial prescribing; MRSA and *C. difficile*; norovirus threat; hospital cleaning and monitoring; *Legionella* control; decontamination of clinical devices; planned maintenance and new builds
7. Surveillance programme and feedback
8. Infection control guidelines
9. Any other business
10. Date and time of next meeting

---

at ward entrances, alcohol gel fixtures where required and organization of a designated Hand Hygiene Day for the Trust. The committee agreed to institute enhanced frequency of hand hygiene monitoring for the hospital, using established World Health Organization guidelines.

Antimicrobial prescribing

Antimicrobial prescribing and consumption are currently key issues for all hospitals. Despite a comprehensive empirical antimicrobial prescribing policy, it was evident that the guidance required updating and auditing. Regular provision of data on antimicrobial consumption for individual departments and wards would assist in targeting inappropriate prescribing. In the absence of the on-site microbiologist, first-line use of broad-spectrum antibiotics, specifically carbapenems and cephalosporins, should be restricted. Quinolone prescribing was also targeted, since junior doctors do not necessarily realize that these agents encourage both MRSA and quinolone-resistant *C. difficile*. There was debate about how such restrictions could be enforced, and it was agreed to implement prescribing penalties following an educational campaign and audit. In addition, stocks of restricted antibiotics should be removed from the wards, except the Intensive Therapy Unit (ITU) and Accident and Emergency, since this would impede inappropriate use out-of-hours.

HAI surveillance

Routine surveillance of key pathogens had identified persistent problems with hospital acquisition of MRSA, multidrug-resistant *Klebsiella* spp. and *C. difficile* among long-term care patients. Lack of isolation rooms compounded control attempts, along with increasing bed occupancy rates in wards for older patients. Current surveillance definitions employed, however, would not identify the origin of acquisition, and it was possible that patients were already carriers before hospital admission, or were actually acquiring HAIs on a busy admissions ward. The group agreed to support an enhanced surveillance programme using national directives in order to identify the most likely site of acquisition. Such data could then be fed back to all relevant staff, including the Trust Board of Directors.

Planning for norovirus

There is a constant threat from norovirus for all healthcare facilities. Control of norovirus outbreaks involves clinical staff, managers, and estates and domestic staff. Pressure on beds pushes managers into opening wards too soon, which can reignite an outbreak in a high-turnover ward. Medical traffic encourages spread to other wards, since nurses can be confined to affected wards but junior medical staff may not necessarily be confined. There also needs to be firm ruling over visitor restrictions when a ward is closed. Ward nurses charged with enforcing the number of visitors should be supported, particularly out of hours. The responsibility for reopening wards following confirmed norovirus needs communication and understanding between infection control and bed managers in the light of recent reports of prolonged shedding from highly persistent strains. Ward closures have a major impact on bed occupancy rates, and can force a hospital to divert patients elsewhere, thus placing pressure on neighbouring hospitals.

Environmental cleaning

Hospital cleanliness remains a priority, since patients frequently complain about their care in so-called 'dirty' hospitals. Lack of guidance on monitoring of surface cleanliness other than visual assessment does not reassure staff or patients that the healthcare environment is truly free from risk of hardy pathogens. Domestic staff are generally compliant with hygiene standards, but there are recurring recruitment difficulties. Managers should support training opportunities for domestic staff, as well as recruit clinical support workers or auxiliary nurses who could take on additional cleaning duties. These would include cleaning clinical equipment, including electrical items. ITU nurses were already routinely targeting clinical equipment, specifically hand-touch sites within the bed space.

Estates issues

Additional items of importance for infection control included review of *Legionella* guidelines and estates practices regarding plumbing incidents and maintenance; review of wash-disinfector rinse water testing and standards; and a formal protocol for inclusion of infection control staff in discussing applications for new buildings and upgrades of facilities throughout the hospital. Without infection control advice, building work and new equipment procurement often cause unforeseen problems relating to environmental risks of infection for patients.

Time was running out for the first meeting of the infection control review group. Discussion had revealed inadequacies and deficiencies in the infection control framework, many of which could be resolved with forward planning, communication and support from senior managers. Lack of isolation facilities in the hospital was potentially the most important item to address for the future, but there were other issues of relevance to consider (Box 3.3). It was agreed to meet in one month's time, with the same members.

Longer-term strategies to support infection control

Given the emphasis on surveillance and audit, the ICNs were stretched to fulfil their routine duties. The review group thus prioritized the appointment of an additional ICN, or secondment of a suitably experienced nurse for surveillance purposes. Audit projects can be supported by appropriate information technology initiatives and access to the

Box 3.3 **Priorities in infection control.**

1. Hand hygiene: compliance monitoring and feedback; education
2. Isolation protocol; guidance for cohorting patients
3. Identification of resources for mandatory surveillance
4. MRSA screening and decontamination protocol
5. Antimicrobial restrictions; reporting; education; policies
6. Decontamination of reusable equipment; monitoring
7. Care of indwelling devices
8. Environmental cleaning; monitoring; training
9. Hospital water supplies: monitoring for *Legionella*
10. Hospital laundry; protocol for management of linen, etc.
11. Infection Control Committee; robust support from senior management
12. Forward planning for outbreak management
13. Education and training in infection control for all staff categories

microbiology laboratory database. There were no easy solutions to the lack of side rooms, but creating additional isolation facilities in certain areas of the hospital (e.g. intensive care) may be feasible. The hospital needed an on-site clinical microbiologist, not only to support pharmacy staff in reducing inappropriate prescribing of antibiotics, but also to manipulate antimicrobial reporting, especially where the organism(s) isolated were more likely to be commensals rather than pathogens.

Conclusion

The main problem for staff responsible for infection control is that an infection incident must occur before resources are identified and control measures put into place. Perhaps *infection prevention* would be a better term to use. It is difficult to estimate the true costs of hospital-acquired infection outwith a defined outbreak situation. Resourcing infection-prevention activities costs a lot less than a hospital outbreak, but this requires vision, capital and a sound evidence base. Much of what is done in the name of infection control is not necessarily based on robust evidence but on 'best practice' or 'informed common sense'. A comprehensive infection-prevention structure requires support from both managers and clinicians in order to maintain appropriate practice and control. This must include involvement of the most senior managers and regular reporting to Trust Boards, since the latter are ultimately responsible for preventing HAI in the hospital.

Further Reading

Dancer SJ. Considering the introduction of universal MRSA screening. *J Hosp Infect* 2008; **69**: 315–20.

Department of Health. Healthcare associated infection. London, UK: NHS. Available at: http://www.dh.gov.uk/en/Publichealth/Healthprotection/Healthcareacquiredinfection/index.htm (accessed 05 08 11).

Fraise AP, Bradley C (eds). *Ayliffe's Control of Healthcare-Associated Infection: A Practical Handbook*. London: Hodder Arnold, 2009.

Heymann DL (ed.). *Control of Communicable Diseases Manual*, 19th edition. Washington DC: American Public Health Association, 2008.

Mehtar S. How to cost and fund an infection control programme. *J Hosp Infect* 1993; **25**: 57–69.

National Institute for Health and Clinical Excellence. Quality standards on healthcare-associated infections in secondary care settings. NICE, 2011. Available at: http://www.nice.org.uk/guidance/phg/advicehealthcareassociatedinfectionsconsultation.jsp (accessed 05 08 11).

World Health Organization. WHO Guidelines on Hand Hygiene in Health Care. Geneva: World Health Organization, 2009.

ANTIBIOTICS

PROBLEM

4 Choosing the Right Antibiotic

Stephanie J. Dancer

Case History

A 66-year-old man was admitted to hospital for increasing problems with urinary retention and recurrent infections. He was admitted to a general medical ward and catheterized whilst awaiting urological opinion. Two days later he developed a urinary tract infection and was started on 2 g ceftriaxone daily by the junior doctor. His symptoms failed to resolve and a catheter specimen of urine was sent for microbiological analysis. This grew an extended spectrum β-lactamase (ESBL)-producing *Klebsiella pneumoniae*, which was resistant to all antibiotics tested except for meropenem. Ceftriaxone was stopped and the patient was prescribed meropenem. One week later he became septic and blood cultures were sent to the laboratory. *K. pneumoniae* was isolated from blood but this isolate was resistant to meropenem. He became colonized with methicillin-resistant *Staphylococcus aureus* (MRSA) and then developed antibiotic-associated diarrhoea, with a stool specimen testing positive for *Clostridium difficile* toxin.

How should this patient be managed?

Why did this patient develop these infections?

What could be done to stop this happening to other patients?

Background

ESBL Gram-negative bacilli are becoming increasingly prevalent in hospitals throughout the world. They are often associated with urinary tract infections but can be isolated from any site. Exposure to sustained antibiotic prescribing has encouraged the appearance of strains that have become increasingly resistant to antibiotics; this began with resistance to the β-lactam agents (e.g. amoxicillin) and the cephalosporins, but has now evolved to include aminoglycosides such as gentamicin, and antibiotics containing β-lactamase inhibitors (e.g. co-amoxiclav and tazobactam). Most ESBL coliforms are also resistant to trimethoprim, nitrofurantoin and quinolones, which means that clinicians are unable to find an oral agent for uncomplicated urinary tract infection. This encourages the use of a parenteral agent such as a carbapenem.

Until now, the carbapenem antibiotics have been the last resort for the treatment of infections caused by multiply resistant coliforms. Now they too are becoming ineffective, as hospital organisms gain additional enzymes, or carbapenemases, capable of hydrolyzing these agents. The term '*extreme drug-resistant*' Gram-negative bacilli has now been introduced in order to differentiate between the ESBL coliforms and new strains resistant to not only carbapenems but to more recent antibiotics, specifically tigecycline. This monotonous and relentless stepwise increase in resistance by these organisms does not bode well for the future, in that patients face infections caused by organisms that are essentially untreatable.

Whilst it is accepted that there is a link between antimicrobial consumption and antimicrobial resistance, it has only recently been appreciated that some antibiotics are better able to encourage resistance than others. Broad-spectrum agents incite the appearance and overgrowth of both naturally resistant organisms and those that have acquired resistance. A simple way of explaining why these agents are more successful at encouraging resistance is to presume that their broad-based effects against a wide variety of organisms kill or inhibit natural commensals on skin or mucosa, thus allowing space for expansion by survivors. These survivors are already resistant to the drug used and take the opportunity to establish themselves as the predominant species. This leads to colonization by organisms usually held in check by the more usual commensals and even infection if the survivors happen to have pathogenic potential. Regarding the patient in this case, it has already been established that third-generation cephalosporins encourage the appearance of ESBL coliforms (Figure 4.1) and, indeed, enterococci, MRSA, *Candida* and *C. difficile*. Carbapenems encourage overgrowth from *Candida*, MRSA and the naturally resistant *Stenotrophomonas maltophilia*.

Management

The patient was placed in a side room after identification of an ESBL *K. pneumoniae* and stayed in isolation for the rest of his time in hospital. Once the results from the blood culture were known, meropenem was stopped and he was started on intravenous fosfomycin (3 g tds) following susceptibility testing. This drug has been used extensively in the past (originally called phosphonomycin) but is not currently listed in the British National Formulary. Prescription should therefore be discussed with the patient, pharmacy and the consultant responsible for the patient. There is a dose adjustment for patients with compromised renal function. Tigecycline was available for use, but the isolate from blood cultures was resistant even to this new antibiotic.

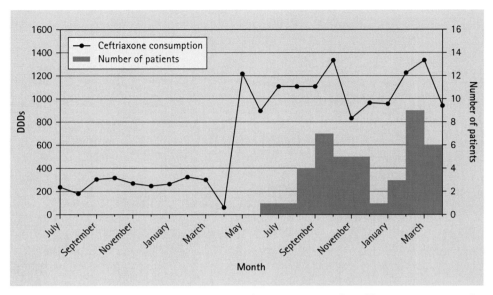

Figure 4.1 Total hospital consumption of ceftriaxone (defined daily doses [DDDs]/1000 patient bed-days) July 2000–April 2002 and number of new patients demonstrating ESBL-producing coliforms (data courtesy of Dr D. Baird).

The patient's urinary catheter was changed after the first dose of fosfomycin. Permanent removal was not an option due to the risk of urinary retention without a catheter *in situ*. Routine swabs had previously identified colonization with MRSA and he was started on a five-day topical clearance regimen. Diarrhoea developed a day later and oral metronidazole was added when the laboratory confirmed the presence of *C. difficile* toxin from stool.

After three days, fosfomycin was stopped and the metronidazole continued for another week. The diarrhoea resolved and the patient appeared to be improving. The *Klebsiella* isolate from blood cultures was sent to a reference facility for further characterization.

Outcome

Three weeks after ESBL septicaemia, the patient became septic once again. His C-reactive protein rose to over 200 mg/l and his white blood cell count was 18×10^9/l. He was given a dose of meropenem during the night by a doctor unaware of the microbiological history. He died the next day. The laboratory isolated ESBL *K. pneumoniae* from blood and a catheter specimen of urine, with both isolates reported as being intermediately resistant to meropenem. No other specimens were taken.

Comment

For each separate infection incident, this patient should have had his urinary catheter changed under appropriate antimicrobial cover, following a full septic screen performed as soon as he became unwell. Treatment with, firstly, ceftriaxone and, secondly, meropenem, encouraged overgrowth from two multiply resistant hospital pathogens and *C. difficile*. It is possible that he was already colonized with ESBL *K. pneumoniae* before he came into hospital, since he had received numerous courses of antibiotics for urinary sepsis whilst resident in the community. In addition, he had acquired *S. maltophilia* whilst in the intensive care unit six months prior to this admission.

Recent Developments

Multidrug resistance has forced clinicians to re-examine drugs used in the past in an attempt to find some active agent with which to treat an infected patient. Fosfomycin is one of these and can be given orally as well as intravenously. Now that ESBL coliforms appear to be moving into the community, an oral formulation precludes hospital admission for parenteral drugs. Another older agent, colistin, is also being used to treat resistant Gram-negative infections, including those caused by *Pseudomonas* spp.

K. pneumoniae from initial blood cultures from the patient was reported to have meropenem minimum inhibitory concentrations (MICs) equal to 8 mg/l, with ertapenem and imipenem MICs of >16 mg/l and equal to 4 mg/l, respectively. The isolate was intermediately resistant to tigecycline (MIC = 2 mg/l). A clover-leaf assay did not detect the presence of a carbapenemase enzyme (see a typical 'clover-leaf' plate; Figure 4.2). It was presumed, although not confirmed, that the mechanism of carbapenem resistance was consistent with permeability changes, including porin loss and upregulated efflux. This type of resistance often masks the phenotypic detection of underlying ESBL activity.

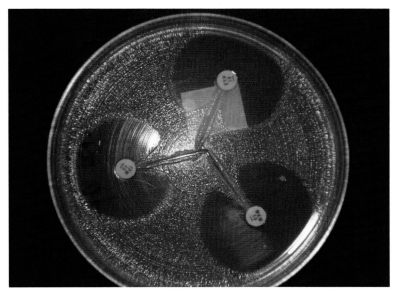

Figure 4.2 Clover-leaf assay. Carbapenem inactivation assays are a rapid and sensitive method for screening carbapenem-resistant isolates. The clover-leaf test is a microbiological assay of carbapenemase activity where the suspect isolate is tested against carbapenem on an agar plate. Altered growth of an indicator strain around the disk is a positive result. One advantage of this test is that enzymes that have very weak carbapenemase activity can be detected by this method. (Photograph courtesy of Dr R. Hill, Health Protection Agency, Colindale, UK.)

Conclusion

Managing an infection caused by a resistant organism can be very difficult. If it remains undetected, the 'wrong' antibiotic will simply make things worse. Even the 'right' antibiotic may do more harm than good if it is given for too short a time or in too low a dose. When an organism proliferates, the signs and symptoms of an infection become more obvious as the rapidly expanding colonies of bacterial cells provoke an inflammatory reaction. Some organisms are able to do a lot more than just increase their numbers. Having found a site and established themselves, they can switch on mechanisms that help them to invade deeper into the tissues. Therefore, giving a patient an inappropriate antibiotic will enhance the virulence of a potential pathogen *in vivo* because it will clear a space for the pathogen and make it easier for it to spread.

It is increasingly important to send appropriate and timely specimens to the laboratory as soon as sepsis is diagnosed. Getting it wrong regarding the choice of antibiotic may kill a vulnerable patient; at best, the patient fails to respond, whilst the organism is given time to evolve its defence mechanisms including virulence, resistance, persistence and spread. In addition, each hospital should have antibiotic policies which guide the clinician towards empirical choices based on narrow-spectrum therapy. Antibiotics such as third-generation cephalosporins and carbapenems should be reserved for specific indications.

Further Reading

Dancer SJ. The problem with cephalosporins. *J Antimicrob Chemother* 2001; **48**: 463–78.

Dancer SJ. Consequences of antimicrobial chemotherapy: overgrowth, resistance and virulence. In: Gould I (ed.). *Antibiotic Policies: Fighting Resistance*. New York: Springer, 2006; 1–15.

Falagas ME, Giannopoulou KP, Kokolakis GN, Rafailidis PI. Fosfomycin: use beyond urinary tract and gastrointestinal infections. *Clin Infect Dis* 2008; **46**: 1069–77.

Findlay J, Hamouda A, Dancer SJ, Amyes S. Rapid acquisition of decreased carbapenem susceptibility in a strain of *Klebsiella pneumoniae* arising during meropenem therapy. *Clin Microbiol Infect* 2011; doi: 10.1111/j.1469-0691.2011.03515.x.

Kollef MH. Appropriate empirical antibacterial therapy for nosocomial infections: getting it right the first time. *Drugs* 2003; **63**: 2157–68.

Paterson DL, Doi Y. A step closer to extreme drug resistance (XDR) in Gram-negative bacilli. *Clin Infect Dis* 2007; **45**: 1179–81.

Queenan AM, Bush K. Carbapenemases: the versatile beta-lactamases. *Clin Microbiol Rev* 2007; **20**: 440–58.

PROBLEM

5 Gentamicin: Issues in Clinical Practice

Alison H. Thomson

Case History

An 82-year-old male with hospital-acquired pneumonia was prescribed a combination of gentamicin and amoxicillin. Gentamicin treatment was initiated according to 'Hartford' guidelines. The patient's creatinine was 66 μmol/l and he weighed 58.6 kg. Estimated glomerular filtration rate (eGFR) was determined as >60 ml/min and creatinine clearance was therefore 63 ml/min (Cockcroft Gault equation):

Creatinine clearance = (140 – 82 [years]) × 58.6 kg × 1.23 [male] /66 mmol/l = 63 ml/min.

An intravenous dose of 400 mg gentamicin (7 mg × 58.6 kg = 410 mg) was given over 30–60 minutes at 10:00 pm. The serum gentamicin concentration at 8:00 am the next morning was 4.3 mg/l and further doses were administered at 10:00 pm that night and the following night. Unfortunately, the first gentamicin dose was given at 4:00 pm, not 10:00 pm; thus, the concentration had been measured at 16 hours and not 10 hours post-dose, as illustrated in Figure 5.1. A further blood sample was therefore withdrawn at 1:00 pm on day four and the gentamicin concentration (15 hours post-dose) was 5 mg/l. Although this was beyond the time limit of the nomogram, it was clearly high and gentamicin was withheld. The concentration in a further sample taken at 8:00 pm was 2.5 mg/l (Figure 5.2).

Why is timing of the measurement of gentamicin concentration important?

What effect does frailty have on the accuracy of the Cockcroft Gault formula and how does this affect gentamicin dosing?

What are the potential adverse effects of gentamicin and how can these be minimized?

Background

In the 1970s and 1980s, gentamicin dosing regimens were driven by 'peak' and 'trough' concentrations following reports that 'cure' was related to peak concentrations above 4 mg/l and toxicity to trough concentrations above 2 mg/l. In the 1990s, 'once daily'

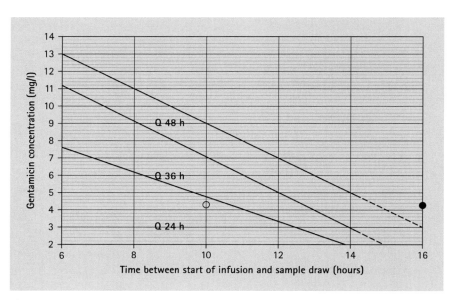

Figure 5.1 Hartford nomogram for determining the gentamicin dosage interval from a blood sample taken 6–14 hours after the dose (adapted with permission from Anaizi 1997). Solid circle represents actual sample time, open circle represents assumed sample time.

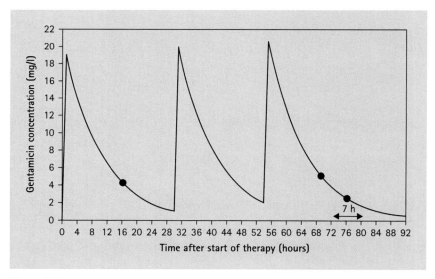

Figure 5.2 Plot of the gentamicin concentration–time profile for the patient. Gentamicin concentration measurements are shown by the solid circles.

regimens emerged in response to new evidence. For example, it was demonstrated that a maximum gentamicin concentration of at least ten times the minimum inhibitory concentration (MIC) of the organism was associated with a clinical response rate of >90%. This compared to a response rate of around 55% if the peak gentamicin concentration was only twice the MIC. Gentamicin dosing is calculated according to 'Hartford' guidelines of 7 mg/kg per 24, 36 or 48 hours, depending on renal function. These guidelines recommend a dose of 7 mg/kg/day to ensure that this high ratio is consistently achieved, even against organisms with MICs up to 2 mg/l. This dose aims to produce a peak concentration around 20 mg/l at the end of a 1 hour infusion and a trough below 0.5 mg/l for at least 4 hours. The guidelines recommend measurement of the serum gentamicin concentration 6–14 hours after the first dose and then plotting the result on the 'Hartford nomogram' to confirm the dosage interval. There is no evidence from clinical studies that efficacy is compromised in patients with such low trough concentrations. The need for such high peaks has been questioned and lower doses, such as 5 mg/kg/day, or fixed doses based on weight and renal function have also been recommended.

Safe and effective use of gentamicin is reliant on accurate dosing and timings for sampling; otherwise, significant misinterpretations will occur. The Cockcroft Gault and eGFR equations assume normal production of creatinine and can sometimes overestimate renal function in frail elderly patients. In this case, the patient is underweight at 58.6 kg (67 kg is the ideal body weight for his height of 172 cm). This is likely to reflect a reduced muscle mass and creatinine production may therefore be lower than normal. If the creatinine measurement itself is low (i.e. below 60 µmol/l), using a minimum value of 60 µmol/l in the equation has been found to give a better indicator of gentamicin dose requirements.

If the measured gentamicin concentration at 6–14 hours is much higher than expected from the creatinine clearance estimate – i.e. it falls into a different dosage interval category – it may indicate a dose or sampling error or an acute decline in renal function. In such cases it is better to confirm that the concentration is <1 mg/l before giving the next dose, rather than simply adjusting the dosage interval according to the guidelines.

When there is uncertainty, the observed decline in the measured gentamicin concentrations can help to determine the appropriate dosage interval. In this case, the concentration halved from 5 mg/l to 2.5 mg/l between 1:00 pm and 8:00 pm on day four, indicating that the elimination half-life was 7 hours. A dosage interval of at least four to five times the elimination half-life (i.e. 36–48 hours in this case) is required to avoid accumulation.

Careful use of gentamicin is important to minimize nephrotoxicity and ototoxicity, which are recognized adverse effects of gentamicin. Due to uptake saturation in the kidney, and potentially inner ear, high peak concentrations do not themselves increase the risk of toxicity. Instead, nephrotoxicity is associated with drug accumulation in the kidney and has been most closely linked to overall exposure, as determined by the area under the concentration–time curve. Consequently, the risk of nephrotoxicity is enhanced by persistently high trough concentrations and a long duration of treatment. Treatment lasting >5–7 days has also been identified as a risk factor for ototoxicity, which is fortunately rare. Unlike nephrotoxicity, ototoxicity is often irreversible and a genetic predisposition has been identified. There is no obvious relationship between ototoxicity and gentamicin concentrations, however, and in the presence of possible hearing or vestibular dysfunction, prescribers cannot be reassured by drug concentrations that are within the therapeutic range. Patients should be monitored closely, especially after seven days of treatment, for any complaints of hearing loss, dizziness, tinnitus or oscillopsia, etc.

Recent Developments

There is compelling evidence to support the use of higher doses of gentamicin with longer dosing intervals. Controversy remains about the exact dose magnitude (5 mg/kg versus 7 mg/kg) and about the dosing interval in patients with renal impairment (36 or 48 hours). To minimize the risk of toxicity, it is advisable to discontinue gentamicin after three days of treatment, if possible.

Conclusion

Overall, safe and effective gentamicin treatment requires close attention to dosage history, interpretation of measured concentrations and clinical response.

Further Reading

Anaizi N. Once-daily dosing of aminoglycosides. A consensus document. *Int J Clin Pharmacol Ther* 1997; **35**: 223–6.

Ariano RE, Zelenitsky SA, Kassum DA. Aminoglycoside-induced vestibular injury: maintaining a sense of balance. *Ann Pharmacother* 2008; **42**: 1282–9.

Cockcroft DW, Gault MH. Prediction of creatinine clearance from serum creatinine. *Nephron* 1976; **16**: 31–41.

Hilmer SN, Tran K, Rubie P *et al.* Gentamicin pharmacokinetics in old age and frailty. *Br J Clin Pharmacol* 2011; **71**: 224–31.

Kirkpatrick CMJ, Duffull SB, Begg EJ. Pharmacokinetics of gentamicin in 957 patients with varying renal function dosed once daily. *Br J Clin Pharmacol* 1999; **47**: 637–43.

Levey AS, Bosch JP, Lewis JB, Greene T, Rogers N, Roth D. A more accurate method to estimate glomerular filtration rate from serum creatinine: a new prediction equation. *Ann Int Med* 1999; **130**: 461–9.

Moore RD, Lietman PS, Smaith CR. Clinical response to aminoglycoside therapy: importance of the ratio of peak concentration to minimal inhibitory concentration. *J Infect Dis* 1987; **155**: 93–9.

Nicolau DP, Freeman CD, Belliveau PP, Nightingale CH, Ross JW, Quintiliani R. Experience with a once-daily aminoglycoside program administered to 2,184 adult patients. *Antimicrob Agents Chemother* 1995; **39**: 650–5.

Rosario M, Thomson AH, Jodrell D, Sharp CA, Elliott HL. Population pharmacokinetics of gentamicin in patients with cancer. *Br J Clin Pharmacol* 1998; **46**: 229–36.

Rybak MJ, Abate BJ, Kang L, Ruffing MJ, Lerner SA, Drusano GL. Prospective evaluation of the effect of an aminoglycoside dosing regimen on rates of observed nephrotoxicity and ototoxicity. *Antimicrob Agents Chemother* 1999; **43**: 1549–55.

Scottish Antimicrobial Prescribing Group. SAPG guidance on gentamicin and vancomycin policies revised. Available at: http://www.scottishmedicines.org.uk/files/SAPG_Guidance_on_gentamicin_and_vancomycin_policies_revised.pdf (accessed 05 08 11).

6 Antibiotic Drug Interactions

Lee Stewart

Case History

A 74-year-old female was admitted to hospital with an infective exacerbation of chronic obstructive pulmonary disease (COPD). She was documented as being allergic to penicillin and her past medical history included COPD, angina and atrial fibrillation. Her inpatient medication chart showed prescriptions for the following:

Digoxin 125 μg each morning*
Warfarin 3 mg each evening*
Simvastatin 20 mg at night*
Co-magaldrox (aluminium hydroxide/magnesium hydroxide) 20 ml when required for indigestion*
Salbutamol 5 mg nebulized four times daily†
Ipratropium bromide 500 μg nebulized four times daily†
Prednisolone 40 mg each morning‡
Clarithromycin 500 mg orally twice daily‡

*Pre-admission medicine, no dose change
†Pre-admission medicine, inhaler changed to nebulized administration on admission
‡New medication started on admission

The patient was concerned about taking clarithromycin, stating that she had been prescribed this before and it had 'upset her other medicines'.

What factors do you need to consider when assessing the significance of drug interactions?

Are drug interactions involving clarithromycin significant in this case?

What is the best approach to management in this case?

Background

A drug interaction occurs when the effect of a specific agent is modified due to the presence of another drug, herbal medicine, food, drink or an environmental chemical.

Drug interactions can be classified as pharmacokinetic interactions (where there is altered drug absorption, distribution, metabolism or elimination) and/or pharmaco-dynamic interactions (where the interaction alters the effect of a drug at its site of action, e.g. by receptor antagonism). The resultant change in drug serum concentration and/or drug effect can cause significant harm to patients both through increased toxicity and treatment failure.

When assessing the potential significance of a drug interaction and deciding on the best management option, a range of factors should be considered. These include:

- Incidence of the interaction and any factors present in the patient that may influence this (e.g. the drug dose, renal/hepatic function, increased susceptibility due to age or other medical conditions). Many interactions show considerable inter-patient variation.
- Potential consequences of the interaction for the patient. The possibility of antibiotic treatment failure in a patient with severe sepsis is unlikely to have an acceptable risk-benefit ratio whereas an interaction resulting in a moderately increased serum concentration of a relatively non-toxic antibiotic may be inconsequential. In some cases (e.g. an antibiotic–oral contraceptive interaction) the temporary loss of a drug's effect may be acceptable for the duration of the antibiotic course (provided appropriate action is taken where necessary; using additional methods of contraception in this case). Particular attention should be paid to the possibility of drug interactions in patients being treated with drugs known to have a high potential for toxicity, or where treatment failure could lead to significant patient harm (e.g. digoxin, warfarin, lithium, antiepileptics, immunosuppressants, anti-infectives). An awareness of common enzyme inducers (e.g. rifampicin, phenytoin, carbamazepine) and common enzyme inhibitors (e.g. macrolides, azole antifungals) may also help to identify potentially serious drug interactions.
- Ease of monitoring for drug efficacy and toxicity. If the impact of the interaction can be assessed relatively easily (e.g. by measuring serum concentrations of the affected drug) then suitable monitoring and dose adjustment may allow the interacting drugs to be used together safely and effectively.
- Timing (onset and offset) of the interaction. This is relevant when deciding on the timescale of monitoring when an interacting drug is added to a medication regimen (and, in the case of an antibiotic, withdrawn).
- Availability of alternative non-interacting drugs and the comparative efficacy and toxicity of these. In some cases switching to an alternative drug may eliminate the interaction altogether; in other cases this may lead to an unacceptable compromise in efficacy or toxicity, leaving no option but to use the interacting drugs.

A variety of information sources are available to help with this type of assessment. Appendix 1 of the British National Formulary (BNF) provides an accessible and comprehensive list of drug interactions, highlighting those likely to have potentially serious consequences. The drug's Summary of Product Characteristics (in most cases these are available online at: http://www.medicines.org.uk/emc/) will contain details of known drug interactions while more detailed information can be obtained by consulting specialist texts (e.g. Stockley's Drug Interactions, which is available via most pharmacists) or by undertaking a literature search.

Clarithromycin and drug interactions

A glance at the BNF Appendix will confirm that clarithromycin (and other macrolides) is involved in a variety of clinically significant drug interactions. For this patient the following are of note:

- Clarithromycin inhibits the cytochrome P450 isoenzyme CYP3A4, which is involved in the metabolism of simvastatin. This interaction increases the serum concentration of simvastatin to cause rhabdomyolysis. Consequently, the concurrent use of simvastatin and clarithromycin is contraindicated.
- Clarithromycin increases the serum concentration of digoxin and this encourages digoxin toxicity. The interaction may be due to clarithromycin increasing the oral bioavailability and reducing renal clearance of digoxin.
- Clarithromycin may increase the effect of warfarin resulting in bleeding. This interaction is subject to considerable inter-patient variation and the mechanism is unclear.

If clarithromycin use was unavoidable (e.g. the only choice for the patient based on culture results) then each of these interactions could be managed to minimize risk. Suspending simvastatin use for the duration of the antibiotic course is a possibility; switching to a statin less likely to interact (e.g. rosuvastatin) would offer an alternative in cases where a prolonged course of clarithromycin was required. The digoxin interaction occurs in most patients and should be managed by monitoring for digoxin toxicity and dose reduction if necessary. Measuring serum digoxin concentrations may help with this, and, depending on the clinical circumstances, pre-emptive dose reduction could be considered if the patient is known to have a serum digoxin concentration close to the upper limit of the target range. Increasing the frequency of anticoagulation monitoring is advisable for all anticoagulated patients receiving antibiotics; here, the warfarin dose should be adjusted to maintain the target international normalized ratio.

It is important to note that the additional monitoring (and potential dose adjustments) required to manage these interactions is equally as important when withdrawing the interacting drug. Given the effort required and the fact that monitoring simply reduces rather than abolishes the risks to the patient, avoiding the interactions altogether would seem to offer a much more satisfactory management solution. In seeking alternatives it should be noted that many antibiotics are involved in drug interactions (Table 6.1).

Table 6.1 Examples of drug interactions involving selected antibacterial agents*		
Antibacterial	**Affected drug(s)**	**Details of interaction**
Aminoglycosides	Vancomycin, amphotericin, ciclosporin, tacrolimus	Combination of nephrotoxic agents increases the risk of nephrotoxicity
	Loop diuretics, vancomycin	Combination of ototoxic agents increases the risk of ototoxicity
Carbapenems	Valproate	Reduced serum concentration of valproate with risk of treatment failure
Daptomycin	Statins, fibrates, ciclosporin	Increased risk of myopathy

continued

Antibacterial	Affected drug(s)	Details of interaction
Fusidic acid	Statins	Increased risk of myopathy
Glycopeptides	Aminoglycosides, amphotericin, ciclosporin, tacrolimus	Combination of nephrotoxic agents increases the risk of nephrotoxicity
	Loop diuretics, aminoglycosides	Combination of ototoxic agents increases the risk of ototoxicity
Isoniazid	Carbamazepine	Increased serum carbamazepine concentration with potential toxicity, increased risk of hepatotoxicity
	Phenytoin	Reduced phenytoin metabolism with increased serum concentration and a risk of toxicity in some patients
Linezolid	Monoamine oxidase inhibitors (MAOIs; e.g. phenelzine, tranylcypromine, isocarboxazid, selegiline, moclobemide)	Additional MAOI effect from linezolid increasing the risk of toxicity
	Antidepressants, lithium	Increased risk of serotonin syndrome
Macrolides	Digoxin	Raised serum digoxin concentration resulting in possible toxicity
	Many drug interactions due to enzyme inhibition (e.g. carbamazepine, pimozide, midazolam, verapamil, colchicine, simvastatin)	Reduced metabolism of the affected drug resulting in increased serum concentration and possible toxicity
Metronidazole	Phenytoin	Possible inhibition of phenytoin metabolism with resultant toxicity
	Alcohol	Possible disulfiram effect (flushing, nausea, vomiting, headache, hypotension)
	Lithium	Possible increase in serum lithium concentration with toxicity
Penicillins	Methotrexate	Reduced methotrexate clearance with possible toxicity
Quinolones	Antacids, iron salts, calcium salts, zinc, strontium ranelate	Complex formation with quinolones in the gut, reducing absorption with potential treatment failure
	Amiodarone	Additive effects from QT interval prolongation increasing the risk of cardiac arrhythmias
	Theophylline	Reduced metabolism of theophylline increasing the risk of toxicity. Possible increased risk of convulsions
Rifamycins	Many drug interactions due to enzyme induction (e.g. clarithromycin, doxycycline, warfarin†, phenytoin, corticosteroids, ciclosporin, contraceptives‡)	Increased metabolism of the affected drug reducing serum concentration with possible treatment failure
Tetracyclines	Antacids, iron salts, calcium salts, zinc, strontium ranelate	Complex formation with tetracyclines in the gut, reducing absorption with potential treatment failure
Trimethoprim/ co-trimoxazole	Amiodarone	Possible increased risk of QT prolongation (with co-trimoxazole)
	Azathioprine, methotrexate	Possible increased risk of haematological toxicity

*The table does not include details of all interactions involving antibacterials and should not be used in place of specialist texts when identifying and managing drug interactions. It provides examples of drug interactions where an antibacterial may influence another drug, but contains few examples of where the antibacterial itself is influenced by another drug. Interactions of this nature are also clinically relevant. †Treatment with any antibacterial should be accompanied by increased monitoring for all patients taking warfarin/other coumarin anticoagulants. ‡Non-enzyme-inducing antibacterial drugs can also interact with contraceptives. Details and advice on management can be found in the BNF.

Management of the patient

Amoxicillin would allow the COPD exacerbation to be treated while avoiding the interactions with digoxin and simvastatin (increased anticoagulation monitoring would still be required). The nature of the patient's penicillin allergy should be established to confirm that penicillin avoidance is really required. In the case of true penicillin allergy then doxycycline would be a good alternative. Again, increased anticoagulation monitoring would be required and the patient's antacid requirement would need to be assessed and reviewed. Antacids containing aluminium or magnesium can reduce the absorption of tetracyclines from the gut significantly through the formation of chelates, resulting in a subtherapeutic serum concentration. If the antacid is required it should be separated from the doxycycline dose by three hours or more to minimize the impact of this interaction.

Recent Developments

Drug interactions are so numerous that it is impossible to memorize them all. Moreover, information on drug interactions is being updated constantly as new drugs are developed and new interactions involving existing drugs are identified. Knowing where to find up-to-date information on interactions is essential when prescribing. In this respect the reference sources detailed are updated regularly and it is important that the current version is consulted when seeking information on drug interactions. Care should be taken when prescribing drugs marketed for only a relatively short period of time; information on potential drug interactions may be limited and some clinically relevant drug interactions may not yet have been identified.

Conclusion

Antibiotics are involved frequently in drug interactions, and while many are of little or no clinical significance, others can lead to significant patient harm through drug toxicity or treatment failure. Avoiding this harm relies on prescribers being alert to the possibility of drug interactions, recognizing drugs and conditions where interactions are likely to be clinically relevant, knowing where to find up-to-date information on drug interactions and taking appropriate action to minimize risk.

Further Reading

Baxter K (ed.). *Stockley's Drug Interactions*. London: Pharmaceutical Press. Available at: http://www.medicinescomplete.com/ (accessed 12 08 11).

Joint Formulary Committee. British National Formulary, 60th edition. London: British Medical Association and Royal Pharmaceutical Society, 2010.

Westphal JF. Macrolide-induced clinically relevant drug interactions with cytochrome P-450A (CYP) 3A4: an update focused on clarithromycin, azithromycin and dirithromycin. *Br J Clin Pharmacol* 2000; **50**: 285–95.

Systems-based Infection

SKIN AND STRUCTURE INFECTIONS

PROBLEM

7 Wound Discharge and Fever

Alan P. Gibb

Case History

A 48-year-old man presented with a three-day history of flu-like illness, with shoulder, neck and thigh pains, but no cough or sore throat. He had noticed groin pain the day before admission, and subsequently groin swelling, redness and difficulty moving. There was no previous history of groin swelling.

He had had an elective laparoscopic cholecystectomy one year previously for biliary colic and was discharged well at that time with a plan to have dressings changed and stitches removed by a community nurse. Over the intervening year he was readmitted to hospital on several occasions for abdominal wall infection, initially at the inferior lateral port site, and subsequently at contiguous sites further down the abdominal wall, requiring drainage on seven occasions. Microbiological investigations of drainage material had yielded methicillin-resistant *Staphylococcus aureus* (MRSA) on one occasion, *Escherichia coli* on another, methicillin-susceptible *Staphylococcus aureus*

(MSSA) on a third, and mixed coliforms on a fourth occasion. He had been treated with a variety of antibiotics for these episodes, some in hospital and some from the general practitioner. He worked as a farm labourer and had a background of Klinefelter syndrome, receiving testosterone implants every four months since age 13.

Why was this man having recurring episodes of apparent infection?

Could we do anything to prevent relapse?

Background

On this latest admission, pulse was 102 beats/min, blood pressure 134/77 mmHg and temperature 38.2°C. There was a firm 3 cm × 3 cm swelling in the groin with no cough impulse. There was erythema over the lower half of the abdomen. The swelling was about 10 cm away from the area of scarring in the upper quadrant related to the previous episodes.

Abdominal X-ray showed the presence of gas in the swollen area. C-reactive protein (CRP) was markedly raised at 165 mg/l and the white blood cell count was 14.2×10^9/l.

Following incision, 7 ml of pus was drained. Gram stain showed Gram-negative bacilli and Gram-positive cocci. Culture yielded mixed coliform organisms, enterococci and anaerobic Gram-negative bacilli.

Initial antibiotic management following incision was with vancomycin and meropenem because of the history of prior MRSA and exposure to multiple antibiotics. His recovery over the next few days was uneventful.

Differential diagnosis

The options considered were:

- Is this an infection, or is it some other process?
- Is it a rare illness (infective or otherwise), or an unusual presentation of a common illness?
- Is the background of Klinefelter syndrome, or the fact that he works on a farm, relevant?

The presentation has many of the features of acute infection (flu-like illness, raised CRP and presence of pus) but this was not supported by the finding of the usual causes of skin sepsis such as *Staphylococcus aureus* or *Streptococcus pyogenes*.

Pyoderma gangrenosum was considered as a possible diagnosis. This inflammatory but non-infective condition is classically associated with inflammatory bowel disease and most often occurs on the shins. Abdominal wall pyoderma gangrenosum is, however, a recognized condition which is difficult to distinguish from acute bacterial infection and has been reported as presenting with an abscess in the groin. It is an important diagnosis to consider as surgical drainage of pyoderma gangrenosum lesions can make them worse, antibiotics do not help and steroids may be the appropriate treatment. Histopathology is not usually helpful in distinguishing pyoderma gangrenosum from infection. A biopsy taken at one of the earlier admissions was reviewed with this in mind, but the features were compatible with pyoderma gangrenosum or infection. In the end the diagnosis of pyoderma gangrenosum was discounted because the drainage wound healed normally.

Underlying gut disease was considered, partly because inflammatory bowel disease is present in about half of patients with pyoderma gangrenosum, but more because of the history of recurring infection following initial biliary surgery, and because the mixture of organisms on this occasion suggested a gut source. Clinical examination and a history of gut function did not suggest any intra-abdominal problem, but a barium enema was performed and no abnormality found.

Further Considerations

Could the Klinefelter syndrome be relevant? The implants received consisted of depot injections into the muscles of the abdominal wall every four months, alternating between the left and right. Over the past year, because of the sepsis on the right side, all injections had been given on the left. We wondered if the presence of lipid deposits in the abdominal wall could predispose to breakdown leading to infection, though we found nothing in the literature on infections of the abdominal wall in Klinefelter syndrome. Sections of the biopsy from previous surgery were stained for fat, but no deposits were seen. We concluded that depot injections were not the cause of the problem.

We also considered the possibility of atypical mycobacterium or fungal infection. There was, however, no evidence of these in biopsy material. We would have expected a persisting chronic problem with such infections rather than the episodes of infection interspersed by periods of normality. Appropriate cultures had not, however, been performed on the specimens and we agreed that they should be done if there was any further recurrence.

The patient works on a farm with sheep and cattle but no exotic animals. There was no history of injury but, on questioning, the patient volunteered that he does frequently climb over barbed wire fences and could have injured himself. Any such injury could easily have introduced faecal organisms from farm animals.

Conclusion

Having considered and rejected a wide range of possibilities, we concluded it most likely that the current episode was due to some unrecognized injury that introduced organisms from the skin into the abdominal wall, and that it is not connected with the previous recurring infections.

There was some concern about whether the post-discharge wound care had been optimal in the past, and we asked that the community nurse took particular care with the wound this time and continued to dress it until completely healed. Antibiotic was stopped after five days and the patient discharged home. There has been no further recurrence in the subsequent year.

This unusual case raised many questions, but in the end we concluded that it was simply a common problem presenting in an unusual context.

Acknowledgement

The author is grateful to Mr Gavin Browning, Consultant Surgeon, for permission to describe this case.

Further Reading

Bhagra S, Arora AS. Fever and an inguinal swelling: pyoderma gangrenosum. *Gut* 2008; **57**: 204, 222.

Brooklyn T, Dunnill G, Probert C. Diagnosis and treatment of pyoderma gangrenosum. *BMJ* 2006; **333**: 181–4.

Lanfranco F, Kamischke A, Zitzmann M, Nieschlag E. Klinefelter's syndrome. *Lancet* 2004; **364**: 273–83.

PROBLEM

8 Animal Bite-related Infection

Marina Morgan

Case History

A 73-year-old lady attended the emergency department nine hours after being bitten on the hand by a stray cat. She complained of severe pain in the wrist and the small puncture wounds seen near the wrist joint were reddened with accompanying lymphangitis and swelling. Despite a temperature of 37.5°C she was systemically well and shortly after the bite took 500 mg of erythromycin supplied by the general practitioner (GP). Her relevant clinical history included severe rheumatoid arthritis, for which she had required multiple joint replacements and steroid therapy. She had also lost her spleen following a road traffic accident 20 years previously but had never taken post-splenectomy penicillin prophylaxis.

What is the likely diagnosis?

How would you investigate this lady?

How would you manage the wound and deal with this infection pending microbiology confirmation?

Background

Although dogs are responsible for 80%–90% of animal bites in the UK, only 36% of bites to the hand become infected. This is due to the mechanical nature of the bite (i.e. shearing trauma), since these comparatively superficial wounds are easily cleaned and debrided. Cat bites have a far higher risk at more than 60% chance of infection. This is partly because of the innocuous appearance of small puncture wounds, which are easily dismissed as insignificant and are difficult to clean. Since bite-related infection of the hand often results in permanent functional impairment, management should be extremely aggressive and thoroughly documented. Failure to recognize a high risk of infection with multiple organisms, particularly *Pasteurella multocida*, and inadequate surgical debridement are major factors associated with poor outcome.

Management options

Patients with animal bites potentially involving a joint should be admitted for surgical exploration, debridement and joint irrigation. In this case, indications for hospital admission include systemic manifestations of infection (temperature and lymphangitis), possible involvement of a joint or tendon, and immunocompromised status (steroids and asplenia).

Three important factors predispose this lady to a high risk of infection. Splenectomy itself confers an increased susceptibility to *Capnocytophaga canimorsus* (Dysgonic Fermenter type 2 or DF2), which presents as an overwhelming meningococcal-like septicaemia. The second factor for infection is steroid therapy and the third is the high-risk nature of the wound itself. The wound is high risk because it is a puncture wound, near the wrist joint, more than 6 hours old and deeply penetrating so cannot be cleaned adequately. Underneath an apparently innocuous wound, underlying nerve and tendon damage and infected joints may be present. Examination under anaesthesia may be necessary, with a thorough washout of any joints involved.

Diagnosis

The most likely organism causing infection in this case is *P. multocida*, literally 'killer of many species'. *P. multocida* is usually isolated from wounds presenting within 12 hours of the bite and has a propensity for metastatic infection involving prosthetic joints and other severe sequelae including brain abscess and osteomyelitis. *P. multocida* septicaemia has an associated mortality of >30%.

Laboratory investigations

Blood cultures are mandatory. Baseline C-reactive protein, a full blood count and electrolyte analysis should be performed. If taken to theatre, joint fluid, deep tissue samples and swabs should be sent for Gram stain and culture.

Initial wound management

- Copious irrigation, using tap water or normal saline
- Removal of foreign bodies (e.g. teeth)
- Thorough wound toilet and debridement, especially if the joint is involved
- Delayed closure if possible
- Elevation and immobilization of the limb
- Antibiotics – see below. Stop the erythromycin immediately
- Send pus and/or a deep wound swab or tissue for culture from infected wounds
- Tetanus prophylaxis

Antimicrobial treatment

Infected bites presenting <12 hours post-injury are particularly likely to be infected with *P. multocida*, which causes an early, intense inflammatory response with considerable tissue involvement. *P. multocida* is inherently resistant to erythromycin and flucloxacillin. Tenosynovitis and erosive synovitis produced by untreated *P. multocida* can lead to irreparable damage requiring amputation.

The GP was quite correct to prescribe antimicrobial prophylaxis for this lady, since she is a patient at high risk of infection, and animal bites should always be taken seriously. She should have been referred immediately for a surgical opinion and debridement, however, in view of the proximity of the bite to the wrist joint.

Erythromycin should never be used as monotherapy for prophylaxis of infection due to animal bites, since it is generally ineffective for Gram-negative organisms and *P. multocida* is almost always resistant. If a patient is allergic to penicillin, then erythromycin plus ciprofloxacin, or doxycycline alone, are better prophylactic options.

Despite the absence of large, double-blinded studies, co-amoxiclav is currently recommended for prophylaxis and early therapy of companion animal bites. Co-amoxiclav covers all the expected oral pathogens present in domestic cats. Where *Pasteurella* spp. and *Bacteroides* spp. predominate, extra cover from agents active against Gram-negative organisms and anaerobes may also be required.

This patient needs aggressive antimicrobial therapy. Not only is this now an established infection, but she has a high risk of prosthetic joint infection with *P. multocida* and even risk of death from septicaemia.

Recent Developments

Methicillin-resistant *Staphylococcus aureus* (MRSA) has been reported in domestic animals, but to date there have been no cases of MRSA infection following a bite and currently there are no guidelines recommending MRSA therapy.

Conclusion

Cat-bite wounds should never be underestimated, and wound management is as important as antimicrobial treatment in preventing infection. This lady underwent wound debridement and *P. multocida* was cultured from both tissues and blood cultures. The joint was not found to be involved so she was treated initially with intravenous co-amoxiclav and oral ciprofloxacin (the latter added due to good tissue penetration). She was discharged home after three days with a further seven days of oral co-amoxiclav and ciprofloxacin. She did not develop secondary prosthetic joint infection and made a good recovery.

Further Reading

Goldstein EJ, Citron DM. Comparative susceptibilities of 173 aerobic and anaerobic bite wound isolates to sparfloxacin, temafloxacin, clarithromycin, and older agents. *Antimicrob Agents Chemother* 1993; **37**: 1150–3.

Holm M, Tärnvik A. Hospitalization due to *Pasteurella multocida*-infected animal bite wounds: correlation with inadequate primary antibiotic medication. *Scand J Infect Dis* 2000; **32**: 181–3.

Keogh S, Callaham M. Bites and injuries inflicted by domestic animals. In: Auerbach PS (ed.). *Wilderness Medicine*, 4th edition. St. Louis: Mosby, 2001; 961–78.

Morgan M, Palmer J. Dog bites. *BMJ* 2007; **334**: 413–17.

Morgan MS. *Capnocytophaga canimorsus* in peripheral blood smears. *J Clin Pathol* 1994; **47**: 681–2.

Morgan MS. Hospital management of animal and human bites. *J Hosp Infect* 2005; **61**: 1–10.

Prodigy guidance. Management of Animal Bites. http://prodigy.clarity.co.uk/bites_human_and_animal/management (accessed 12 08 11).

Rohrich RJ. Man's best friend revisited: who's watching the children? *Plast Reconstr Surg* 1999; **103**: 2067–8.

Smith MR, Walker A, Brenchley J. Barking up the wrong tree? A survey of dog bite wound management. *Emerg Med J* 2003; **20**: 253–5.

Talan DA, Citron DM, Abrahamian FM, Moran GJ, Goldstein EJC. Bacteriologic analysis of infected cat and dog bites. *N Engl J Med* 1999; **340**: 85–92.

PROBLEM

9 Community-acquired MRSA

Marina Morgan

Case History

A 19-year-old student was admitted for the fourth time in six weeks for incision and drainage (I&D) of a recurrent large abscess, this time located in the left groin. The lesion demonstrated early necrosis at the centre and was incredibly tender. He had healing wounds from three previous I&Ds – post-auricular, right buttock and left calf – and there was an early lesion appearing on the right calf. He had just completed a seven-day course of oral flucloxacillin (500 mg qds) from his general practitioner (GP), who had excluded diabetes mellitus. In the referral note, the GP had wondered whether this case was due to an 'unusual foreign infection', since the patient had recently returned from an athletics tour of the USA. Following I&D, pus was sent for culture and methicillin-resistant *Staphylococcus aureus* (MRSA) was isolated. Unusually for a UK MRSA isolate, it was susceptible to erythromycin, clindamycin, fusidic acid, doxycycline, co-trimoxazole, gentamicin, ciprofloxacin and rifampicin.

What is the likely diagnosis?

How would you investigate this man?

What general advice would you give for dealing with this infection pending microbiology confirmation?

Background

The most likely clinical diagnosis is infection with a Panton-Valentine leukocidin (PVL)-producing *Staphylococcus aureus*. PVL destroys defensive polymorphs, resulting in bacterial survival and recurrent skin sepsis, with compensatory overproduction of leukocytes. Recurrent skin and soft tissue infection (SSTI) is the classical presentation of PVL disease. Developing further abscesses whilst taking adequate doses of flucloxacillin alerts the physician to the possibility that the *S. aureus* is methicillin resistant (i.e. MRSA).

Clinically, it is impossible to differentiate between PVL-producing community-acquired MRSA (CA-MRSA) and methicillin-susceptible *S. aureus* (MSSA). CA-MRSA can be defined as MRSA isolated from patients in an outpatient or community setting with no previous history of MRSA infection or colonization, hospitalization, surgery, dialysis or residence in a long-term care facility within one year of MRSA culture. Apart from intrinsic resistance to flucloxacillin, early CA-MRSA strains were relatively susceptible to antibiotics. However, ciprofloxacin-, tetracycline- and even mupirocin-resistant CA-MRSA strains are now emerging. A tender lesion with an ulcerating/necrotic centre reminiscent of a 'spider bite' (a phenomenon not uncommon in the USA) suggests CA-MRSA. CA-MRSA causes 60%–70% of SSTIs presenting to emergency departments in the USA.

The face, neck and buttocks account for nearly 50% of the distribution of lesions. Unsurprisingly, CA-MRSA spreads easily in overcrowded living conditions, especially when personal items are shared. Hence, athletes who pluck or shave body hair, or use communal saunas, towels or baths with other athletes, are at greater risk of acquiring CA-MRSA. PVL-producing strains have a predilection for exposed collagen, so wounds or rough skin will be more likely to harbour PVL-positive strains.

Following colonization, the risk of invasive infection varies. In a small religious community 14% of residents became infected, whereas in a marine training facility the actual infection rate was 37% for CA-MRSA. This rate fell to only 3% for those already colonized with non-PVL-producing MSSA.

Debate about when to use antimicrobials for CA-MRSA continues. Treatment with I&D alone was reported to be successful in 85% of patients, especially with lesions with an abscess diameter of less than 5 cm. Another trial reported a small but significant increase in treatment failures with inadequate antimicrobial therapy. The choice of antimicrobial depends on susceptibilities. Most UK CA-MRSA remains susceptible to ciprofloxacin, clindamycin, trimethoprim and mupirocin.

Management options

Recurrent abscesses warranting I&D are unusual in a fit young man. History-taking should concentrate on acquisition risks, particularly sporting activities and close personal contact with colleagues with boils/abscesses. The microbiology department should be asked to refer the isolate for PVL testing and, if positive, the local Health Protection Unit should be informed in case epidemiological investigations are necessary (Figure 9.1).

If the patient presents with spreading cellulitis, blood cultures, a full blood count and C-reactive protein (CRP) should be taken. Suspicion of PVL infection should alert clinicians to the risk of more serious invasive infection such as haematogenous necrotizing pneumonia, purpura fulminans or osteomyelitis. Pending confirmation of PVL status, appropriate infection control measures should be instigated where possible, including isolation and notification of the hospital infection control team.

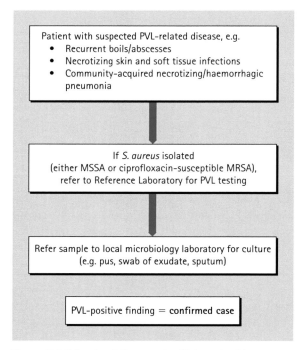

Figure 9.1 PVL-related disease: microbiology algorithm.

I&D of small abscesses in the absence of cellulitis may suffice but, where indicated, oral doxycycline (100 mg twelve-hourly) or fusidic acid (500 mg eight-hourly) or tri-methoprim (200 mg twelve-hourly) together with rifampicin (300 mg twelve-hourly) is recommended. Serious infections justify empirical parenteral vancomycin, teicoplanin, daptomycin or linezolid. Patients with systemic illness need intravenous antibiotics, preferably agents blocking toxin production such as clindamycin or linezolid.

Since broken skin harbours staphylococci, decolonization may be difficult but, given recurrent lesions and spreading cellulitis, systemic antimicrobials and simultaneous decolonization are justified. Whilst unlikely to eradicate carriage until the lesion has healed, decolonization will reduce the risk of spread to family/close contacts and auto-infection of other sites following trauma. Routine hospital MRSA decolonization is rec-ommended, namely chlorhexidine 4% or triclosan 2% body washes in combination with nasal mupirocin for five days (see the information leaflet available from the Department of Health/Health Protection Agency website).

Patients should be warned about the likely diagnosis of CA-MRSA; the risk of trans-mission to close contacts; the importance of hygiene, particularly hand hygiene; the need to keep lesions covered; and the fact that any contacts with symptoms should seek medi-cal advice. They should not attend any sporting facilities (gyms, swimming pools, saunas) until lesions resolve and the skin has completely healed.

With a CRP of 120 mg/l and spreading cellulitis, along with a history of recent travel to the USA where clindamycin-resistant MRSA is increasing, he was empirically treated with oral rifampicin 300 mg bd and linezolid 600 mg bd. Later, when clindamycin susceptibility was confirmed, therapy was changed to oral clindamycin 450 mg qds plus oral fusidic acid 500 mg tds for a total of two weeks. Decolonization was started during the first night of admission. He was successfully cleared of MRSA carriage after two decolonization treatments and remains symptom free.

Recent Developments

CA-MRSA is becoming more resistant to antibiotics and is now spreading in hospitals. Multiresistant strains may necessitate expensive agents such as daptomycin or tigecycline. New glycopeptides and topical antimicrobials are undergoing clinical trials for infections caused by these strains.

Conclusion

CA-MRSA spread in the community and hospitals will blur the margins between hospital and community strains. Awareness and culturing of recurrent lesions are essential for early recognition.

Further Reading

Hota B, Ellenbogen C, Hayden MK, Aroutcheva A, Rice TW, Weinstein RA. Community-associated methicillin-resistant *Staphylococcus aureus* skin and soft tissue infections at a public hospital: do public housing and incarceration amplify transmission? *Arch Int Med* 2007; **167**: 1026–33.

Lewis D, Campbell R, Day C *et al.* The diagnosis and management of PVL-associated *Staphylococcus aureus* infections (PVL-SA) in England: report of the PVL subgroup of the Steering Group Healthcare Associated Infection, 2008. Available at: http://www.hpa.org.uk/PVL-SA_FinalGuidance.pdf (accessed 12 08 11).

Moran GJ, Krishnadasan A, Gorwitz RJ *et al.* Methicillin-resistant *S. aureus* infections among patients in the emergency department. *New Engl J Med* 2006; **355**: 666–74.

Nathwani D, Morgan M, Masterton RG *et al.* Guidelines for UK practice for the diagnosis and management of methicillin-resistant *Staphylococcus aureus* (MRSA) infections presenting in the community. *J Antimicrob Chemother* 2008; **61**: 976–94.

RESPIRATORY TRACT INFECTIONS

PROBLEM

10 Severe Community-acquired Pneumonia

Gavin Barlow

Case History

A 66-year-old woman was admitted to hospital with a two-week history of chills and diarrhoea. On examination she was lucid and had the following observations: respiratory rate 22 breaths/min, blood pressure 107/59 mmHg and pulse oximetry 90% (on air). The blood urea was 8.2 mmol/l. The acute medical team diagnosed gastroenteritis and she was prescribed intravenous fluids. She was transferred to another ward two days later where the doctor ordered a chest radiograph. This showed pneumonia in the right middle and lower zones. Antibiotic therapy was prescribed and oxygen initiated. Although the diarrhoea improved, the patient remained unwell after four days.

What is the cause of this patient's diarrhoea?

How should the doctors assess the severity of this patient's illness?

How should the doctors decide which antibiotic therapy to use?

What are the potential causes for the lack of improvement?

Background

Diagnosis

Pneumonia is difficult to diagnose without a chest radiograph and it is not unusual for patients to present with non-respiratory symptoms such as diarrhoea. This emphasizes the importance of always performing an early chest radiograph for patients admitted to hospital with a febrile illness and/or acute respiratory symptoms, and for the elderly with non-specific deterioration. Chest radiographs may be interpreted incorrectly or be of suboptimal quality in the acutely unwell patient and may occasionally even appear normal in patients shown to have pneumonia by subsequent imaging. When there is a strong clinical suspicion of severe community-acquired pneumonia (CAP), initial therapy should be commenced prior to chest radiography. The low pulse oximetry in the patient described was a clue to her underlying illness, although this can occur in sepsis of non-respiratory origin.

There is no evidence that a clinical entity of 'atypical pneumonia' exists. A microbiological diagnosis is made in a minority of patients hospitalized with CAP; detailed microbiological investigation should therefore be targeted at severe CAP. Panton-Valentine leukocidin (PVL) toxin-producing community-acquired *Staphylococcus aureus* strains occasionally cause devastating pneumonia in fit young adults, which is characterized by temperature >39°C, respiratory rate >40 breaths/min, tachycardia >140 beats/min, hypotension and haemoptysis; such cases should be discussed immediately with a critical care specialist as ventilatory support is likely to be required. Rapid sputum microscopy and culture is necessary to confirm aetiology and determine methicillin resistance. Advice should be sought from an infection specialist.

Severity assessment

The British Thoracic Society recommends the CURB-65 score for the assessment of illness severity in CAP. The acronym stands for:

- **C**onfusion: in a patient who is not normally confused (a mental state questionnaire [MSQ] score of ≤8/10) or a two-point fall in MSQ from baseline (if known) or a clear history of deterioration
- **U**rea >7 mmol/l (if available)
- **R**espiratory rate ≥30 breaths/min
- **B**lood pressure: systolic <90 mmHg and/or diastolic ≤60 mmHg
- Age ≥65 years

One point is scored for each of the above criteria present with a maximum score of 5. The score divides patients into severe and non-severe categories (Figure 10.1). When the blood urea is not available, CRB-65 has been shown to stratify patients similarly to CURB-65. CURB-65 is moderately good at detecting patients with CAP who subsequently die. It may, however, occasionally underestimate severity in the young and is poor at detecting those who subsequently require admission to critical care units. It is therefore important to apply clinical judgement, including assessment of sepsis criteria and severity, and then confirm using the patient's score. CURB-65 has not been validated as a 'track and trigger' score; many acute medical units use early warning scores, but these have been shown to perform less well than CURB-65 at initial assessment.

Linking severity assessment with initial therapy

Due to concerns over *Clostridium difficile*-associated diarrhoea and the emergence and spread of antibiotic-resistant bacteria, the intensity of antibiotic therapy should be guided by severity. It has been consistently shown that patients with a CURB-65 score of 0 or 1 have low mortality, regardless of antibiotics, and it is therefore safe to manage these patients as outpatients (Figure 10.1). Patients with a CURB-65 score of 2 are at higher risk so an antibiotic regimen tailored to the potential causative organism(s) is recommended (Figure 10.1). Patients with a CURB-65 score of 3 or more are at high risk and have most to lose by inadequate treatment; antibiotic therapy should cover all of the common and less common causes (Figure 10.1).

Assessment of oxygenation and hydration status and early review by critical care are also important, particularly in severe CAP; patients should be managed according to the Surviving Sepsis Campaign principles.

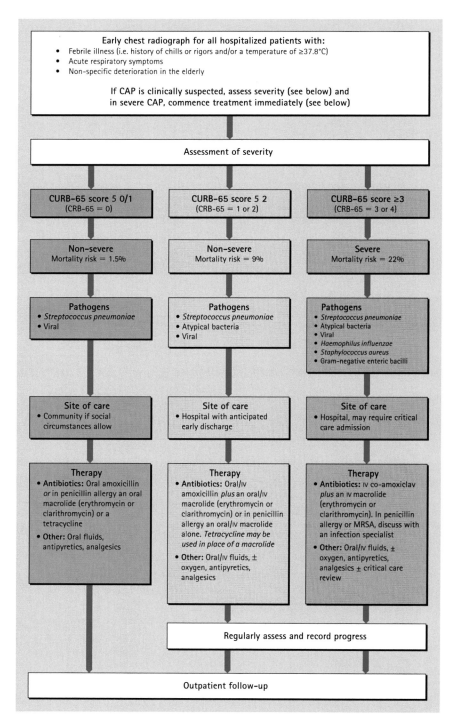

Figure 10.1 The key components of care in community-acquired pneumonia. ɪᴠ, intravenous.

Assessment of the poorly responding patient

Antibiotic resistance is often a concern but it is still unusual among common chest pathogens in the UK. Infection may be due to a virus or, if the patient has initially received β-lactam monotherapy, due to an 'atypical' pneumonia pathogen, all of which can cause pneumonia alone or as co-pathogens. Patients sometimes develop hospital-acquired infection, which can confuse the original diagnosis. Antibiotic concentrations in the lung may be suboptimal due to under-dosing or poor tissue penetration, although this is unlikely when standard doses of β-lactams are used. Poor compliance may also be a possibility, due to patient refusal or intolerance or lack of intravenous access. Important and common reasons that must be excluded are:

1 Empyema, parapneumonic effusion or lung abscess
2 Additional pathologies (e.g. lung cancer) or alternative diagnoses (e.g. pulmonary embolism, pulmonary oedema, etc.).

The patient described in this chapter underwent a repeat chest radiograph, which showed a new pleural effusion; this was drained. A subsequent computed tomography scan showed both pneumonia and a previously undiagnosed lung tumour. It should also be remembered that deterioration often represents the natural history of that patient's infection rather than true failure.

Recent Developments

Various biomarkers appear to be able to assist in severity assessment and antibiotic decision making in CAP. In moderate to severe CAP, prednisolone was shown to reduce the duration of symptoms. Combination therapy (i.e. a β-lactam antibiotic plus a macrolide) was shown to improve survival in patients admitted to the intensive care unit with CAP and shock. Such developments are interesting and a step forward, but should not yet be considered part of standard practice. In the future, the microbiological diagnosis of CAP is likely to be quicker and more accurate through the use of molecular methods.

Conclusion

Making an early diagnosis followed by immediate severity assessment and, in severe CAP, rapid administration of antibiotics and supportive care are the key elements in the optimal management of CAP. Patients who are not improving at 48 hours should be assessed carefully by an experienced physician.

Further Reading

Barlow G, Nathwani D, Davey P. The CURB65 pneumonia severity score outperforms generic sepsis and early warning scores in predicting mortality in community-acquired pneumonia. *Thorax* 2007; **62**: 253–9.

British Thoracic Society Standards of Care Committee. BTS guidelines for the management of community-acquired pneumonia in adults. *Thorax* 2001; **56**(Suppl 4):1–64.

Charles PG, Wolfe R, Whitby M *et al.* SMART-COP: a tool for predicting the need for intensive respiratory or vasopressor support in community-acquired pneumonia. *Clin Infect Dis* 2008; **47**: 375–84.

Christ-Crain M, Stolz D, Bingisser R *et al.* Procalcitonin guidance of antibiotic therapy in community-acquired pneumonia: a randomized trial. *Am J Respir Crit Care Med* 2006; **174**: 84–93.

Dellinger RP, Carlet JM, Masur H *et al.* Surviving Sepsis Campaign guidelines for management of severe sepsis and septic shock. *Crit Care Med* 2004; **32**: 858–73.

Mikami K, Suzuki M, Kitagawa H *et al.* Efficacy of corticosteroids in the treatment of community-acquired pneumonia requiring hospitalization. *Lung* 2007; **185**: 249–55.

Rodríguez A, Mendia A, Sirvent JM *et al.* Combination antibiotic therapy improves survival in patients with community-acquired pneumonia and shock. *Crit Care Med* 2007; **35**: 1493–8.

PROBLEM

11 Multidrug-resistant Tuberculosis

Helena White

Case History

A 47-year-old unemployed white British man with a background of heavy alcohol intake and treatment for tuberculosis (TB) presented with a four-month history of haemoptysis, weight loss and fever. Markedly malnourished, his chest X-ray revealed cavitations in both upper lobes, and sputum microscopy showed numerous acid-fast bacilli. He had had limited contact with health services and had frequently moved accommodation. A diagnosis of multidrug-resistant TB was considered.

Which factors increase a person's risk of developing drug-resistant TB?

What are the definitions of the terms 'multidrug-resistant TB' and 'extensively drug-resistant TB'?

How is a diagnosis of drug-resistant TB established?

What management strategies need to be employed in the treatment of drug-resistant disease?

Background

Tuberculosis remains one of the major global health challenges. Incidence has increased as a result of the human immunodeficiency virus (HIV)/acquired immune deficiency syndrome pandemic, and population growth and increased migration have contributed towards the current UK incidence. Reactivated TB in elderly British individuals is now outnumbered by infection in young foreign migrants.

Multidrug-resistant TB (MDRTB) is defined as resistance to both first-line drugs, rifampicin and isoniazid. Extensively drug-resistant TB (XDRTB) is MDRTB with additional resistance to any fluoroquinolone plus one second-line injectable aminoglycoside: amikacin, kanamycin or capreomycin. In comparison with fully susceptible strains, MDRTB and XDRTB cause more severe disease, with increased mortality, present greater challenges in planning and administering treatment and incur greater treatment costs.

The global scale

Across the world, 5% of newly diagnosed TB is MDRTB, amounting to half a million new cases per year. In the UK, MDRTB accounts for 1.2% of cases. To date, 45 countries have reported cases of XDRTB, including one in the UK (Figure 11.1).

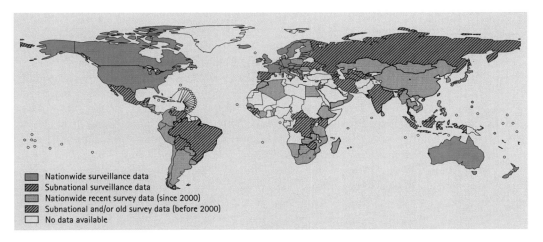

Nationwide surveillance data
Subnational surveillance data
Nationwide recent survey data (since 2000)
Subnational and/or old survey data (before 2000)
No data available

Figure 11.1 Countries that have reported at least one case of XDRTB by the end of 2010 (from www.who. int/tb/challenges/mdr/drs_maps_feb2011.pdf).

Risk factors for drug resistance

Poor adherence to therapy confers the highest risk for drug resistance, with homelessness, substance misuse and poverty compounding the risk in vulnerable individuals. In accordance with other chronic disease management, healthcare providers have a responsibility to ensure that patients at risk of poor compliance receive adequate support, including access to directly observed therapy (DOT), the use of key workers to engage with patients and increased financial and housing support.

Co-infection with HIV and foreign birth, particularly in sub-Saharan Africa and the Indian subcontinent, are other risk factors for drug-resistant TB in the UK.

Across the world, drug resistance emerges wherever drugs are used indiscriminately and without adequate monitoring, particularly when availability of pharmaceuticals is unregulated. Countries most affected are those where HIV burden is high, and where management systems for disease control are weak.

A risk assessment for drug resistance should be undertaken whenever TB is diagnosed, with special vigilance for relapsed and imported disease.

Diagnosis

Sputum examination for mycobacteria underpins all TB programmes, but routine culture and susceptibility testing are beyond the resources of many poor or conflict-torn countries.

In developed economies, solid-medium culture has been superseded by liquid culture, encouraging more rapid growth of organisms for susceptibility testing. Molecular probes differentiating between *Mycobacterium tuberculosis* complex and atypical mycobacteria may be helpful in some instances. Molecular probes for rifampicin and isoniazid resistance enable drug resistance to be rapidly detected. Early liaison with reference laboratories is essential to ensure appropriate use of these resources.

Management

An immediate priority for patients with suspected drug-resistant TB is their accommodation in negative-pressure isolation facilities to minimize transmission to patients and healthcare workers. When unavailable, single-room nursing and personal protection with appropriate fitted masks are mandatory. In the UK, management should be undertaken only by experienced clinicians, particularly when HIV coexists and drug interactions are common and complex. Notification to public health authorities and urgent contact tracing must be undertaken. Sputum should be sent to a reference laboratory for resistance testing. Nutritional management, HIV testing and measures to ensure adherence are essential aspects of future care.

Box 11.1 Drug management of drug–resistant tuberculosis (adapted with permission from World Health Organization. Guidelines for the programmatic management of drug–resistant tuberculosis. WHO/HTM/TB/2006.361. WHO, 2006).

Treatment regimens for MDRTB should:

- Take into account drugs taken during previous TB episodes
- Take into account known local or outbreak resistance patterns
- Comprise at least four drugs with certain or almost certain effectiveness against the strain; more if susceptibility is unknown or there is questionable effectiveness of an agent, or extensive bilateral pulmonary disease is present
- Include an injectable agent for the first six months of treatment
- Provide a total treatment duration of a minimum of 18 months
- Provide drugs that are given on at least six days per week
- Be DOT-based to ensure compliance

The World Health Organization has outlined the management principles of MDRTB and XDRTB (Box 11.1). Combination therapy is based on the strain antibiogram or, in endemic areas, according to local epidemiological patterns. Standardized protocols in some countries reduce the need for specialized laboratory services and simplify procedures such as procurement of second-line agents. The formation of the UK National MDRTB Group in 2008 enables discussion between experts regarding the management of individual cases.

Recent Developments

 Gamma-interferon assays to facilitate earlier diagnosis of latent infection are used increasingly by developed nations, and molecular polymerase chain reaction typing methods assist in the identification of strains in outbreak settings. New anti-TB drugs and vaccine trials are emerging as potential new strategies, but public health focus is aimed at strengthening existing measures through The Global Plan to Stop TB 2006–2015 partnership.

Conclusion

 Multidrug-resistant TB is increasing globally and is a major public health and clinical challenge. Priorities for TB control and management (including multidrug-resistant disease) include: dedicated funds; reinforcement of health infrastructure, including laboratory susceptibility testing; wider availability of HIV treatment; improved availability of second-line anti-TB drugs; and experienced and adequately trained personnel.

Further Reading

Chapman ALN. Antituberculosis drug resistance: new global data on an emerging global emergency. *Clin Med* 2008; **8**: 478–9.

Health Protection Agency. Tuberculosis in the UK: Annual report on tuberculosis surveillance in the UK 2008. London: Health Protection Agency Centre for Infections, 2008.

National Collaborating Centre for Chronic Conditions. Tuberculosis: clinical diagnosis and management of tuberculosis, and measures for its prevention and control. London: Royal College of Physicians, 2006.

Stop TB Partnership. The Global Plan to Stop TB 2006–2015. Available from: http://www.stoptb.org/global/plan/ (accessed 13 09 11).

van Deutekom H, Supply P, de Haas PEW *et al*. Molecular typing of *Mycobacterium tuberculosis* by mycobacterial interspersed repetitive unit-variable-number tandem repeat analysis, a more accurate method for identifying epidemiological links between patients with tuberculosis. *J Clin Microbiol* 2005; **43**: 4473–9.

World Health Organization. Guidelines for the programmatic management of drug-resistant tuberculosis. WHO/HTM/TB/2006.361. WHO, 2006.

World Health Organization. The WHO/IUATLD Global Project on Anti-Tuberculosis Drug Resistance Surveillance. Anti-tuberculosis drug resistance in the world. Report no. 4. WHO/HTM/TB/2008.394. WHO, 2008.

12 Suspected Q Fever

Paul Robertson

Case History

A 55-year-old farmer with a history of moderate mitral regurgitation attended his local medical receiving unit. He described an abrupt illness with four days of fever, headache, myalgia, vomiting and breathlessness that had begun two weeks after lambing season. His temperature was 39.1°C and respiratory rate was 28 breaths/min, but there were no other abnormalities found on examination. Blood investigations showed a mild transaminitis and elevated C-reactive protein, but his full blood count, urea and electrolyte panel, and plasma glucose were normal. A chest X-ray showed right mid-zone consolidation. Based on his epidemiological risk factors, Q fever was suspected.

When should a diagnosis of Q fever be suspected and how should it be confirmed?

Who is at risk of chronic Q fever? How can it be prevented?

How should you treat the different presentations of Q fever?

Background

Q fever is a zoonotic infection caused by *Coxiella burnetii*, an intracellular pathogen. The annual incidence in the UK is 1–2 cases per million, but it is much more common in southern Europe and Australia. Although *C. burnetii* can infect many animals, the most common sources of human infection are sheep and cattle. Spontaneous abortion may be the only indication of infection. Those working with livestock, such as vets, farmers and abattoir workers, are most at risk. A spore-like form of *C. burnetii* can survive in dust and be easily spread by air currents over several miles. Several large community outbreaks have occurred in the UK, likely due to wind-borne spread from nearby farmland. *C. burnetii* is highly infectious, with fewer than ten inhaled organisms capable of causing disease.

Human infection with *C. burnetii* can cause both an acute and a chronic form of disease. Acute Q fever is seasonal, usually occurring in the late spring and summer following lambing season. After an incubation period of 1–3 weeks, it causes an abrupt, non-specific febrile illness in around 40% of those infected, the remainder being asymptomatic. Pneumonia, hepatitis and, more rarely, meningo-encephalitis are more serious manifestations. Around 5% of those with acute Q fever require hospitalization, but death is exceedingly rare. Acute Q fever is diagnosed serologically by detecting a rising titre to phase II immunoglobulin M (IgM) antibodies. The 'phase' of *C. burnetii* refers to a change in cell surface lipopolysaccharide that is associated with changing biological properties. Phase II organisms easily enter cells in acute infection but are rapidly killed, whereas phase I forms enter cells slowly but can survive with phagolysosomes to cause persistent infection, also known as chronic Q fever. This antigenic change can be detected serologically with the development of persistently elevated anti-phase I immunoglobulin G (IgG) antibody titres (1:800 or greater). The most common manifestation of chronic Q fever is endocarditis (85% of cases), although the presentation is typically indolent with fever and vegetations on echocardiography often absent initially. Vascular graft infection and osteomyelitis can also occur. Regardless of the site of infection, chronic Q fever presents insidiously over several months with multiple non-specific symptoms such as sweats, weight loss and fatigue. Without a prior history of Q fever it can be difficult to consider. It should always be excluded where an unexplained chronic illness develops in the context of pre-existing valvular heart disease or prosthetic valves. Despite improving antimicrobial therapy, chronic Q fever remains difficult to cure and carries significant mortality and morbidity. Post-Q fever syndrome is poorly understood but thought to represent a post-infective syndrome characterized by fatigue, myalgia and arthralgia, among other symptoms. Its cause is unknown and there is no evidence that repeated or prolonged antimicrobial therapy improves symptoms.

Management options

The management of Q fever is shown in Figure 12.1. This patient has non-severe community-acquired pneumonia (CAP). The occupational exposure to livestock and occurrence during lambing season raise the possibility of Q fever as the cause. Although high fever, multisystem symptoms and deranged liver function tests are common in acute Q fever, they are not diagnostic. The diagnosis can be confirmed by paired serological testing for *C. burnetii* phase II IgM – a single negative titre during the illness is insufficient to exclude the diagnosis. A period of diagnostic uncertainty is inevitable while results are awaited. Short courses of single antimicrobial agents during acute Q fever can reduce the duration of symptoms, but are unlikely to reduce the risk of chronic Q fever. Recovery without specific antibiotic treatment is common. No randomized controlled trial (RCT) has compared efficacy of antimicrobial agents or assessed the ideal duration of antimicrobials in acute Q fever. Most guidance suggests 2–3 weeks of doxycycline 100 mg bd, although macrolides and quinolones are also likely to be effective. This patient should be treated according to standard protocols for CAP, such as the British Thoracic Society guidelines, with amoxicillin and a macrolide. Given the strong epidemiological risk, it would be reasonable to replace the macrolide antibiotic with doxycycline.

Further Considerations

A vital part of managing acute Q fever is identifying those who are at increased risk of chronic Q fever. Chronic Q fever complicates 1%–2% of cases of acute Q fever, but certain groups, including those who are immunosuppressed, pregnant or who have prosthetic vascular grafts, are at higher risk. The single biggest risk factor for chronic infection is pre-existing valvular heart disease; 30%–40% of those with valvular heart disease who are infected with *C. burnetii* will develop chronic Q fever. This risk can be reduced by giving a prolonged course of doxycycline 100 mg bd and hydroxychloroquine 200 mg bd. The optimal duration of preventative therapy has not been determined but it should be

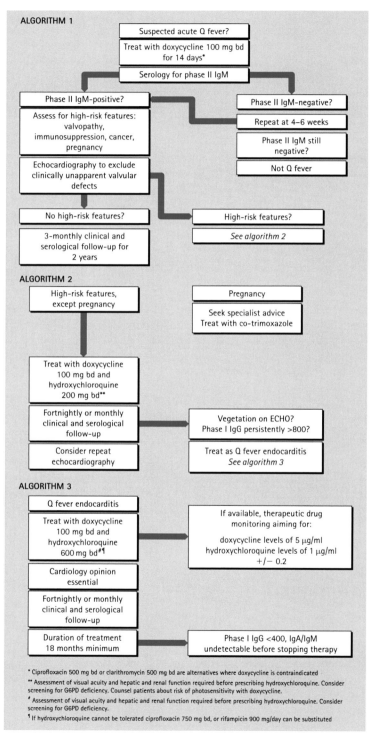

ALGORITHM 1

Suspected acute Q fever?

Treat with doxycycline 100 mg bd for 14 days*

Serology for phase II IgM

Phase II IgM-positive?

Assess for high-risk features: valvopathy, immunosuppression, cancer, pregnancy

Echocardiography to exclude clinically unapparent valvular defects

Phase II IgM-negative?

Repeat at 4–6 weeks

Phase II IgM still negative?

Not Q fever

No high-risk features?

3-monthly clinical and serological follow-up for 2 years

High-risk features?

See algorithm 2

ALGORITHM 2

High-risk features, except pregnancy

Pregnancy

Seek specialist advice Treat with co-trimoxazole

Treat with doxycycline 100 mg bd and hydroxychloroquine 200 mg bd**

Fortnightly or monthly clinical and serological follow-up

Consider repeat echocardiography

Vegetation on ECHO? Phase I IgG persistently >800?

Treat as Q fever endocarditis See algorithm 3

ALGORITHM 3

Q fever endocarditis

Treat with doxycycline 100 mg bd and hydroxychloroquine 600 mg bd#¶

Cardiology opinion essential

Fortnightly or monthly clinical and serological follow-up

Duration of treatment 18 months minimum

If available, therapeutic drug monitoring aiming for:

doxycycline levels of 5 µg/ml hydroxychloroquine levels of 1 µg/ml +/- 0.2

Phase I IgG <400, IgA/IgM undetectable before stopping therapy

* Ciprofloxacin 500 mg bd or clarithromycin 500 mg bd are alternatives where doxycycline is contraindicated

** Assessment of visual acuity and hepatic and renal function required before prescribing hydroxychloroquine. Consider screening for G6PD deficiency. Counsel patients about risk of photosensitivity with doxycycline.

Assessment of visual acuity and hepatic and renal function required before prescribing hydroxychloroquine. Consider screening for G6PD deficiency.

¶ If hydroxychloroquine cannot be tolerated ciprofloxacin 750 mg bd, or rifampicin 900 mg/day can be substituted

Figure 12.1 Management of Q fever. ECHO, echocardiography; G6PD, glucose 6-phosphate dehydrogenase.

given for several months if tolerated. Echocardiography is recommended in all patients with acute Q fever to exclude pre-existing valvular heart disease, particularly bicuspid aortic valve or mitral valve prolapse that may not be apparent on clinical examination. All patients with acute Q fever should be offered serological follow-up to allow identification of chronic Q fever at an early stage.

There is also a lack of RCT evidence to guide choice or duration of therapy for chronic Q fever. As few antibiotics kill *Coxiella* within the acidic phagolysosome, cure is difficult. Hydroxychloroquine alkalizes the phagolysosome, which enables doxycycline to have bacteriocidal activity. Therefore, the most effective current treatment is doxycycline combined with hydroxychloroquine. This combination is superior to doxycycline and a fluoroquinolone, which in turn is more effective than doxycycline monotherapy. Monitoring hydroxychloroquine levels is prudent to ensure adequate dosing. Treatment should be for a minimum of 18 months and continued until phase I IgM levels are undetectable. Where doxycycline and hydroxychloroquine is not tolerated or is contraindicated, there is no clear preferred second-line therapy. Quinolones, co-trimoxazole and rifampicin have all been used with some degree of success. Lifelong therapy may be necessary when any of these agents are used.

Conclusion

Q fever is suspected in this case of CAP because of seasonality and occupational risk. Samples should be sent for *C. burnetii* phase II IgM testing at presentation and after 4–6 weeks. Until the diagnosis is confirmed, treatment with amoxicillin and a macrolide or doxycycline should be given. The patient's valvular heart disease places him at high risk of developing chronic Q fever. On serologically confirming the diagnosis of Q fever, he should be treated with doxycycline and hydroxychloroquine for at least one month, ideally longer if tolerated. He will require regular serological, clinical and echocardiographic follow-up to ensure endocarditis does not develop.

Further Reading

Fenollar F, Fournier P-E, Carrieri MP, Habib G, Messana T, Raoult D. Risk factors and prevention of Q fever endocarditis. *Clin Infect Dis* 2001; **33**: 312–16.

Habib G, Hoen B, Tornos P *et al.*; ESC Committee for Practice Guidelines. Guidelines on the prevention, diagnosis, and treatment of infective endocarditis (new version 2009): the Task Force on the Prevention, Diagnosis, and Treatment of Infective Endocarditis of the European Society of Cardiology (ESC). Endorsed by the European Society of Clinical Microbiology and Infectious Diseases (ESCMID) and the International Society of Chemotherapy (ISC) for Infection and Cancer. *Eur Heart J* 2009; **30**: 2369–413.

Healy B, Llewelyn MB, Westmoreland D, Lloyd G, Brown N. The value of follow-up after acute Q fever infection. *J Infect* 2006; **52**: 109–12.

Raoult D, Houpikian P, Tissot Dupont H, Riss JM, Arditi-Djiane J, Brouqui P. Treatment of Q fever endocarditis: comparison of 2 regimens containing doxycycline and ofloxacin or hydroxychloroquine. *Arch Intern Med* 1999; **159**: 167–73.

Raoult D, Marrie TJ, Mege JL. Natural history and pathophysiology of Q fever. *Lancet Infect Dis* 2005; **5**: 219–26.

GENITOURINARY INFECTION

PROBLEM

13 Management of Acute Uncomplicated Pyelonephritis

Beryl Oppenheim

Case History

A 37-year-old woman presented to an accident and emergency department. She complained to the assessing doctor that she had had severe right loin pain and had been experiencing fevers and shivering for the past 24 hours. She had felt nauseous and had vomited on two occasions. She had also noticed burning on passing urine. On examination she was found to be pyrexial, with a temperature of 39.5°C, and had a tachycardia of 120 beats/min and a blood pressure of 100/60 mmHg. She had tenderness around the right flank.

What is the clinical diagnosis?

What investigations should the doctor perform?

How should this patient be managed?

Background

Acute pyelonephritis is a clinical condition characterized by severe loin pain or tenderness, fever and rigors, and often nausea and vomiting. It can occur with or without symptoms of dysuria such as urinary frequency and burning on micturition. It is essentially an infection of the urinary tract which involves the kidney. The condition can range in severity from a mild to moderate infection which responds to simple antibiotic therapy, to a severe infection with multiorgan failure. Complications include scarring of the kidneys and impairment of renal function. Acute pyelonephritis is extremely common, with a recent population-based study in the USA noting an overall rate of 15–17 cases per 10 000 women and the annual societal cost of treatment of the condition being estimated at greater than $2 billion. This chapter will address only acute uncomplicated pyelonephritis in non-pregnant adult women and does not include the scope of management in pregnancy, children and males.

Diagnosis

The usual work-up for an infected patient, such as full blood count, urea and electrolytes and C-reactive protein, is required to assist in assessing severity and the need for supportive treatment. Blood cultures are of value in severe infection and, although of lower yield in mild to moderate cases, should still be considered in hospitalized, particularly elderly patients, in whom the systemic inflammatory response may be blunted.

The most important microbiological investigation is urinalysis. Dipstick testing will reveal nitrites and leukocyte esterase but it is essential to send a properly collected mid-stream urine specimen for culture so that an accurate identification of the pathogen and its antimicrobial susceptibility can be obtained. The majority of cases of acute pyelonephritis reveal $>10^5$ organisms/ml, but it is generally recommended that $>10^4$ organisms/ml is reported.

Important and reversible predisposing factors to acute pyelonephritis, particularly obstruction, can be excluded by an ultrasound examination of the abdomen, possibly accompanied by a plain X-ray. If these suggest relevant pathology then further imaging may be required.

Infecting organisms

The major infecting organisms for acute pyelonephritis are the same as those that cause lower urinary tract infection, with *Escherichia coli* predominating and other Gram-negative organisms such as *Klebsiella* spp. and *Proteus* spp. also important. Local susceptibility patterns should be available for reference.

Management

An algorithm for the management of acute pyelonephritis is shown in Figure 13.1. Despite the fact that acute pyelonephritis is a commonly encountered infection, there are relatively few evidence-based studies on which to base recommendations for treatment. In addition, two recent developments affecting management of infection, in the UK at any rate, limit the applicability of a number of these studies. These developments include recent concerns over severe infections due to *Clostridium difficile* and the constraints these place on the prescribing of cephalosporins and fluoroquinolones; and the increasing rates of resistance of Gram-negative bacteria, particularly *E. coli*, to both of these antibiotic classes. In England, resistance to ciprofloxacin in *E. coli* strains causing bloodstream infections has been increasing continuously, from 9% in 2002 to 23% in 2006.

Requirement for hospitalization

Many cases of mild to moderate severity acute pyelonephritis can be managed with oral antimicrobial treatment as an outpatient. Patients with severe disease and evidence of sepsis must clearly be managed in hospital with relevant monitoring and supportive treatment, but it is also important to consider initial hospitalization for those patients with nausea or vomiting who may be unable to tolerate oral antibiotics in the early stages of treatment.

Antimicrobial treatment

Choice of agent and route of administration

Initial choice of antimicrobial will be guided by departmental protocols which are informed by local susceptibility patterns, and this choice may need to be modified when results of urine culture become available. Choice of initial therapy may also be influenced

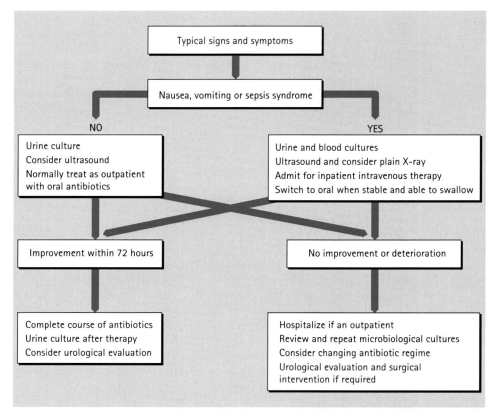

Figure 13.1 Algorithm for the management of acute pyelonephritis (adapted with permission from Engel & Schaeffer, 1998).

by the requirement to avoid those antimicrobials thought to specifically predispose to the development of *C. difficile* infection (CDI). In addition, a number of studies recommend the use of trimethoprim-sulfamethoxazole in areas where resistance is low but this agent is limited in usage in the UK due to concerns over toxicity. Possible initial choices of oral antibiotics could include co-amoxiclav or ciprofloxacin, with the proviso that they are used with caution. For patients requiring intravenous therapy alternative agents may include gentamicin and/or piperacillin-tazobactam, or a second- or third-generation cephalosporin, again bearing in mind possible risks of CDI.

Patients who are haemodynamically unstable with signs of sepsis require initial intravenous therapy. Similarly, anyone with nausea and vomiting should also be started on parenteral antibiotics. If these situations are excluded, however, there does not seem to be any particular benefit from treating all cases of acute pyelonephritis with intravenous antibiotics. Oral agents, or switch therapy with sequential conversion of intravenous to oral as soon as the patient is clinically stable, appear to be effective in both treating the initial infection and preventing long-term damage to the kidneys.

Duration of therapy

Once again, there are few studies clarifying the optimal duration of treatment. Studies have shown the adequacy of a seven-day course of ciprofloxacin, but this has not necessarily been the case for other agents where longer duration of treatment, up to 14 days, has been recommended.

Failure to respond to therapy

The first step should be to review any positive cultures and ensure that the infecting organism is susceptible to the chosen agent. If this is the case, or no organism was identified, then further imaging including a computed tomography scan may be appropriate to exclude any obstruction or abscess formation. In cases where no urological abnormality can be found it may be that the initial choice of agent was inappropriate or that the duration was insufficient, so an alternative agent should be considered. If the patient responds, then a minimum of 14 days' treatment should be given. If an obvious cause for the failure is found on imaging, then surgical treatment may be required to correct the obstruction or drain an abscess.

Requirement for follow-up investigations

Most experts recommend a follow-up urine specimen for culture to ensure bacteriological cure, although it is unclear whether this is done routinely or to assist with further management. No other investigations are required in women with first episodes of infection, but recurrent infection or infection in other patient groups is normally an indication for further investigation.

Recent Developments

There are three important factors which will determine future treatment and prophylaxis options for urinary tract infection:

1   The increasing prevalence of antibiotic resistance, particularly of extended spectrum β-lactamase-producing Gram-negative organisms.
2   The rising vulnerable, elderly population in hospitals and the community, whose risk of CDI is strongly associated with prescribing of agents typically relied on in the management of urinary tract infection, notably cephalosporins, quinolones and extended spectrum β-lactam antibiotics.
3   The lack of new antibiotics in the developmental pipeline, particularly those with good bioavailability and activity against resistant Gram-negative organisms.

Conclusion

Many questions remain regarding the optimal management of pyelonephritis. Choice of agent, route of administration and duration of therapy should be carefully considered for individual patients, taking into account the risk of drug resistance and relative risk of CDI. Locally agreed and regularly updated management guidelines that address such issues are essential.

Further Reading

Blossom DB, McDonald LC. The challenges posed by reemerging *Clostridium difficile* infection. *Clin Infect Dis* 2007; **45**: 222–7.

Czaja CA, Scholes D, Hooton TM, Stamm WE. Population-based epidemiologic analysis of acute pyelonephritis. *Clin Infect Dis* 2007; **45**; 273–80.

Engel JD, Schaeffer AJ. Evaluation of and antimicrobial therapy for recurrent urinary tract infections in women. *Urol Clin North Am* 1998; **25**: 685–701.

Health Protection Agency. Antimicrobial resistance and prescribing in England, Wales and Northern Ireland, 2008. London: Health Protection Agency, 2008. Available at: http://www.hpa.org.uk/web/HPAwebFile/HPAweb_C/1216798080469 (accessed 13 09 11).

Lautenbach E. Finding the path of least antimicrobial resistance in pyelonephritis. *Clin Infect Dis* 2008; **47**: 1159–61.

Livermore DM, Hope R, Brick G, Lillie M, Reynolds R. Non-susceptibility trends among Enterobacteriaceae from bacteraemias in the UK and Ireland, 2001–06. *J Antimicrob Chemother* 2008; **62**(Suppl 2): ii41–54.

Pohl A. Modes of administration of antibiotics for symptomatic severe urinary tract infections. *Cochrane Database Syst Rev* 2007; CD003237.

Talan DA, Krishnadasan A, Abrahamian FM, Stamm WE, Moran GJ. Prevalence and risk factor analysis of trimethoprim-sulfamethoxazole- and fluoroquinolone-resistant *Escherichia coli* infection among emergency department patients with pyelonephritis. *Clin Infect Dis* 2008; **47**: 1150–8.

PROBLEM

14 Complicated Urinary Tract Infection with ESBL-producing *E. coli*

Achyut Guleri, Rashmi Sharma, Michael Przybylo

Case History

A 75-year-old male with a two-year history of vascular dementia was admitted with a three-day history of episodic confusion, agitation and urinary incontinence. Three weeks earlier, following a two-day history of dysuria, a mid-stream specimen of urine (MSSU) had grown *Escherichia coli* resistant to trimethoprim, amoxicillin and cefalexin but susceptible to nitrofurantoin. The report mentioned 'ESBL positive'. The patient had responded to a five-day course of nitrofurantoin for cystitis. Past medical history included hypertension, ischaemic heart disease and dyslipidaemia, and current medication was aspirin, ramipril, bisoprolol, furosemide, isosorbide mononitrate and simvastatin.

On examination the patient was agitated and dehydrated; temperature was 38.3°C, blood pressure 90/45 mmHg and heart rate 110 beats/min. Palpation of his left flank revealed marked tenderness. Mental status examination showed the patient to be confused in person, place and time. Urine dipstick testing was positive for leukocytes, nitrites and protein. There was a peripheral neutrophilia and C-reactive protein was 150 mg/l. Urea and creatinine were elevated, and a plain radiograph and computed tomography (CT) scan of the renal tract revealed a left renal calculus (Figure 14.1).

Blood and MSSU samples were sent for culture and intravenous (IV) fluids and co-amoxiclav IV 1.2 g every eight hours (q8h) were initiated for suspected urosepsis. Gentamicin was withheld due to acute kidney injury. Several hours after admission, he became anuric, acidotic and severely hypotensive. After further fluid resuscitation, haemofiltration was commenced.

After 12 hours, incubation blood cultures revealed Gram-negative bacilli in both bottles, and leukocytes and organisms were seen in the urine. Meropenem 1 g q12h (based on haemofiltration dose) was commenced and the patient was moved to a single room with barrier nursing precautions.

Subsequently, both urine and blood cultures grew an extended spectrum β-lactamase (ESBL)-positive *E. coli* with a similar antibiogram to that from the initial urine sample sent by the general practitioner. Clinical improvement was observed and the dose of meropenem was increased to q8h as renal function normalized. Subsequent follow-up in urology included investigation and treatment for kidney stones.

Why was the initial choice of co-amoxiclav for urosepsis suboptimal?

What are ESBLs?

Why did this patient require barrier nursing and a single room?

What are the different therapeutic options for treating ESBL-associated infections?

Background

Urinary tract infections (UTIs) can range from asymptomatic bacteriuria to pyelonephritis complicated with renal abscesses and severe sepsis with life-threatening bacteraemia. Elderly patients often have asymptomatic bacteriuria that does not require treatment unless they are symptomatic. Reactive use of antibiotics in response to MSSU results in elderly patients can lead to selection of multidrug-resistant bacteria. A history of urinary symptoms (dysuria, frequency, urgency and flank pain) is suggestive of UTI and urine dipstick testing offers a reasonable method of diagnosis (with the exception of catheterized subjects). Urine cultures are recommended for: (i) those with suspected acute pyelonephritis; (ii) any suspected UTI in men; (iii) symptoms that do not resolve or recur within 2–4 weeks after the completion of treatment; and (iv) pregnant women and those

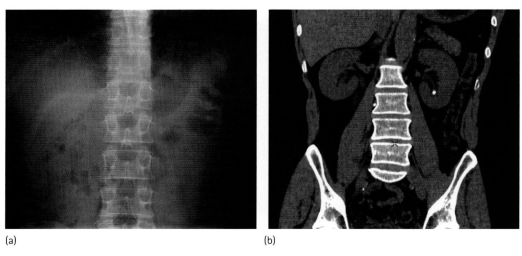

(a)   (b)

Figure 14.1(a) Plain abdominal X-ray and **(b)** coronal CT scan showing left lower pole renal stone (courtesy of Des Alcorn, Consultant Radiologist, Gartnavel General Hospital, Glasgow).

who present with atypical symptoms. Acute pyelonephritis is suggested by flank pain, nausea and vomiting, fever (>38°C), or costovertebral angle tenderness, and it can occur in the absence of cystitis symptoms. Urine and, in patients with sepsis syndrome, blood for culture must be taken before any antimicrobial therapy is started. Evaluation of the upper urinary tract with ultrasound should be performed to rule out urinary obstruction or renal stone disease. Additional investigations/procedures should be guided by the urologists if the patient remains febrile after 72 hours of treatment. Empirical broad-spectrum antibiotics (as per local policy) should be de-escalated once susceptibilities are available.

The patient was promptly and correctly diagnosed and managed but antibiotic choice was suboptimal. It is extremely important that antibiotic choice is informed by previous culture reports as well as local empirical prescribing guidelines. Previous isolation of an ESBL-producing organism may not be apparent at the time of the admission but the history of previous UTIs and the presence of severe sepsis should encourage broader-spectrum empirical therapy. Local knowledge of the rate of ESBL-producing organisms is also invaluable. If gentamicin is absolutely contraindicated, an alternative agent with ESBL activity should be selected with a view to rapid de-escalation if a more susceptible organism is isolated. Risk of *Clostridium difficile* infection, presence of methicillin-resistant *Staphylococcus aureus* carriage and presence of β-lactam allergy are other important considerations in empirical antibiotic choice.

ESBLs, or extended spectrum β-lactamases, are bacterial enzymes in *E. coli* and other members of Enterobacteriaceae that hydrolyze and confer resistance to all penicillins, cephalosporins and monobactams (except cephamycins, pivmecillinam and temocillin). These organisms may also simultaneously be resistant to aminoglycosides, quinolones, co-trimoxazole-trimethoprim and chloramphenicol.

Consultation with a microbiologist can help optimize the management and outcomes of patients with ESBL-associated infections both in primary care as well as within hospital. Preventing the spread of ESBL-producing organisms within hospitals is essential, particularly as infections may be devastating in compromised patients. Stringent hand hygiene compliance, barrier nursing and, if possible, single-room nursing helps prevent cross-transmission of the multidrug-resistant bacteria from patients to staff, other patients and the environment. Involvement of the infection prevention and control team is vital in this regard.

While carbapenems (meropenem, imipenem, doripenem or ertapenem) are the empirical agents of choice for treating severe ESBL-associated infections, there may be further options based on results of urine culture and susceptibility testing (Table 14.1). Oral options for uncomplicated or lower UTI may include trimethoprim, nitrofurantoin, pivmecillinam, fosfomycin or ciprofloxacin, and parenteral options may include piperacillin-tazobactam, gentamicin, amikacin, co-trimoxazole or temocillin. Tigecycline has activity against ESBL-producing organisms but is not indicated in UTIs and bacter-

Table 14.1 Antimicrobials potentially with activity versus ESBL–producing organisms

Drug name	Class	Mechanism of action	Dose	Route	Warnings
Nitrofurantoin	Nitrofurans	Damages cellular DNA	50–100 mg qds	Oral	Simple cystitis use only; long-term prophylaxis associated with pulmonary toxicity
Trimethoprim	Dihydrofolate reductase inhibitor	Inhibits synthesis of tetrahydrofolic acid	200 mg bd	Oral	Long-term usage may cause blood disorders
Ciprofloxacin	Fluoroquinolones	DNA gyrase inhibitor	500 mg bd	Oral	*C. difficile* infection risk, tendinitis
Fosfomycin		Inhibits bacterial cell wall biogenesis	3 g single dose	Oral	
Pivmecillinam	Penicillin	Inhibits cell wall synthesis	400 mg loading following 200 mg tds	Oral	
Temocillin	Penicillin	Inhibits cell wall synthesis	1–2 g bd	IV	
Co-trimoxazole	Dihydrofolate reductase inhibitor–sulfamethoxazole combination	Inhibits synthesis of tetrahydrofolic acid	960 mg bd	IV	Sulpha allergy (rash and fever)
Ertapenem	Carbapenem	Inhibits cell wall synthesis	1 g od	IV	Seizure in renal failure
Imipenem/cilastatin	Carbapenem	Inhibits cell wall synthesis	1–2 g in 3–4 divided doses	IV	Seizure in renal failure
Meropenem	Carbapenem	Inhibits cell wall synthesis	500–1000 mg tds	IV	
Doripenem	Carbapenem	Inhibits cell wall synthesis	500 mg tds	IV	
Tigecycline*	Glycylcycline	30S ribosome protein synthesis inhibitor	100 mg loading following 50 mg bd	IV	Diarrhoea, nausea and vomiting
Colistin	Polymyxin	Solubilizing bacterial membrane	1–2 million units tds	IV	Neurotoxicity, nephrotoxicity

*Tigecycline is NOT indicated in treatment of urinary tract infections and bacteraemia.

aemia due to ineffective concentrations in the blood or urinary tract. Intravenous colistin may be an option in a penicillin-anaphylactic patient with an ESBL-producing organism resistant to all other options. Optimum duration of therapy and the timing of an IV-to-oral switch depends on the site and severity of the infection. In general, parenteral therapy for between five and seven days is preferred for patients with bacteraemia. Oral therapy may be continued for up to one month in male patients with associated prostatitis where relapse is common. Optimal therapy should be agreed with a microbiologist.

Recent Developments

ESBL-associated infections are increasing in prevalence in hospitals in the UK and globally. Inevitably this will lead to difficult decisions regarding empirical and targeted antibiotic choice. When should carbapenem antibiotics be advocated as routine empirical therapy in patients with community-onset sepsis? If widespread empirical use of carbapenems is advocated then it is essential that rapid de-escalation policies are in place to ensure prudent use of this valuable resource. Overuse of carbapenems will encourage further resistance. Carbapenemase-producing organisms are already well established in some parts of the world and even extremely drug-resistant organisms are emerging. The current antimicrobial armamentarium is inadequate for this new public health threat.

Conclusion

Urinary tract infection is one of the most common types of infection seen in both hospitals and the community. Current treatment options are diminishing due to the rapid spread of resistant strains. Sending a specimen of urine to the laboratory before antimicrobial therapy begins will furnish useful information should the causative pathogen display multiple antibiotic resistances. Patients infected with these strains should be subject to strict infection control protocol in hospitals.

Further Reading

Falagas ME, Karageorgopoulos DE. Extended-spectrum beta-lactamase-producing organisms. *J Hosp Infect* 2009; **73**: 345–54.

Health Protection Agency. Investigations into multi-drug resistant ESBL-producing *Escherichia coli* strains causing infections in England. London: Health Protection Agency, 2005. Available at: http://www.hpa.org.uk/web/HPAwebFile/HPAweb_C/1274090495083 (accessed 13 09 11).

Lahey Clinic. β-Lactamase classification and amino acid sequences for TEM, SHV and OXA extended-spectrum and inhibitor resistant enzymes. Available at: http://www.lahey.org/Studies/ (accessed 13 09 11).

15 Proctitis: Focus on Lymphogranuloma Venereum

Andrew J. Winter

Case History

A 28-year-old man was referred by his general practitioner with several weeks of painful defecation and constipation. He had not responded to simple measures such as haemorrhoid cream and laxatives. He had significant weight loss. On closer questioning he reported some transient lymphadenopathy, sore throat and rash three months previously. Proctoscopy revealed an intensely inflamed rectum with a mucopurulent discharge and an evident stricture. Biopsies were non-specific and he failed to improve with application of local rectal steroid. Fortunately at this stage a sexual history was obtained; the patient reported receptive anal sex at a London gay-scene venue four months previously. A rectal swab was positive for *Chlamydia trachomatis* by a nucleic acid amplification test (NAAT).

Why is a sexual history important in this case?

How should his rectal *Chlamydia trachomatis* be managed?

What other infections may this person be at risk of?

Background

Taking a careful sexual history in this case was the key to diagnosis. Several sexually transmitted infections (STIs) can present to the generalist in unusual ways, including sexually acquired proctitis (as here), secondary syphilis, symptomatic human immuno-deficiency virus (HIV) infection, sexually reactive arthritis and disseminated gonococcal infection. Obtaining a good sexual history requires privacy, tact and good rapport-building skills. All practitioners should be able to enquire in a non-judgemental fashion about recent and lifetime sexual risk, which should include gender of sexual partners (do not assume this until you have asked: "Was that with a male or female partner?"), type of sexual activity (e.g. receptive anal sex, protected or unprotected), and country of origin of sexual partners. Men who have sex with men (MSM) may be initially reluctant to disclose MSM activity, particularly if they are not 'out' to family or friends, or are concerned about the practitioner's response. Some patients may not appreciate that symptoms could be related to an STI, or may undervalue the risk of certain activities. Some patients with known HIV infection may be afraid or embarrassed to disclose this in a general medical setting. It is worth specifically asking if someone has previously been diagnosed HIV-positive.

The differential diagnosis of sexually acquired proctitis includes rectal chlamydia, gonorrhoea, herpes and primary syphilis. Routine work-up should exclude all of these, ideally by molecular amplification tests, which are superior to culture tests, as well as including stool examination for *Shigella* and *Salmonella*. Ideally, patients should be referred to a genitourinary medicine service for direct microscopic examination of rectal slides by Gram stain, and dark ground examination of any suspected chancre.

In 2004, several urban centres in Europe, including the UK, reported a significant rise in proctitis due to lymphogranuloma venereum (LGV) affecting predominantly MSM. LGV is caused by lymphotrophic serovars of *Chlamydia trachomatis* (L1–L3) which are highly invasive compared to non-LGV biovars where infection is limited to squamo-columnar cells. In 'classical' (bubonic) LGV, genital infection leads to a transient ulcer followed by significant lymphadenopathy, and can result in the 'genito-ano-rectal' syndrome of extensive pelvic and rectal inflammation, fistulae and genital elephantiasis. In the recent outbreaks, the typical presentation is of early intense proctocolitis with prominent symptoms of tenesmus and constipation and rapid stricture formation (Figure 15.1). Some cases have pronounced systemic symptoms of weight loss and fatigue. Histology of rectal biopsies is easy to confuse with Crohn's disease. Most cases are in Caucasian MSM of whom around 75% are co-infected with HIV and 15%–20% with hepatitis C. Putative risk factors include fisting and enema use, as well as receptive anal intercourse, but the reason for the recent resurgence in cases remains a mystery. In many cases diagnosis is delayed with both patient and physician failing to appreciate the significance of the symptoms and signs, or mistaking them for malignancy or severe inflammatory bowel disease. Figure 15.2 shows the current approach to diagnosing LGV in the UK, where there have been over 700 definite cases reported to August 2008.

In this case, as soon as the positive *C. trachomatis* test is received he requires treatment with doxycycline 100 mg twice-daily orally for three weeks. The laboratory should be asked to refer the rectal sample to the relevant reference centre for LGV testing by real-time polymerase chain reaction (PCR). Epidemiological data may be requested for national

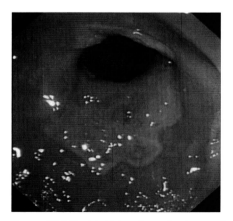

Figure 15.1 Rectal stricture formation in sexually acquired lymphogranuloma venereum infection (courtesy of Dr R. F. McKee) (*see inside front cover for colour version*).

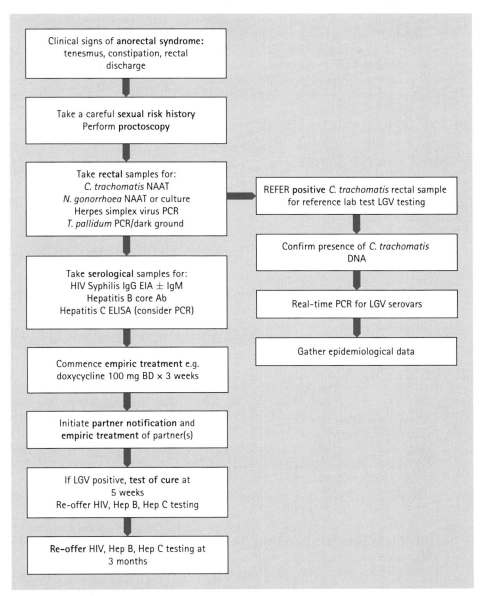

Figure 15.2 Flowchart for investigation and management of suspected sexually acquired proctitis. Ab, antibody; EIA, enzyme immunoassay; ELISA, enzyme-linked immunosorbent assay; Hep B, hepatitis B; Hep C, hepatitis C; PCR, polymerase chain reaction.

surveillance. The patient here also has symptoms suspicious of HIV seroconversion or secondary syphilis. Consent must be obtained for urgent HIV and syphilis serological tests, along with hepatitis B and hepatitis C markers. Excluding sexual infection at other anatomical sites is required (e.g. urine testing for *Chlamydia*/gonorrhoea NAAT, throat culture or NAAT testing for gonorrhoea). Follow-up with a coloproctologist should be arranged in view of the risk of stricture formation. Hepatitis B vaccination should be commenced if not previously completed. Partner notification and epidemiological treatment of ongoing partners are essential to avoid reinfection, and are best undertaken by a skilled sexual health adviser in a genitourinary medicine department. Test of cure for chlamydia remains recommended in LGV cases due to the paucity of data on antibiotic effectiveness, but should be at least five weeks after treatment completion. At three months, retesting for HIV, syphilis and hepatitis C should be offered if initially negative.

Recent Developments

The resurgence of sexually acquired proctitis triggered a rapid evolution in testing methodology. Molecular (NAAT) testing for chlamydia and, more recently, gonorrhoea is now well established in STI testing settings. Although manufacturers have not validated their tests on non-genital specimens, there is now excellent evidence that selected commercial NAAT tests provide good predictive value at these sites. Standard NAAT tests cannot distinguish LGV chlamydial serovars from non-LGV (B and D–K) serovars without expensive and time-consuming DNA sequencing. Newer real-time PCR methods allow for fast sample turnaround and detection of mixed infections, and several methods are now published that utilize molecular differences between LGV and non-LGV serovars to distinguish them. These can even be applied to paraffin-embedded material (rectal and lymph node biopsies). It is unlikely that these methods will become commercially available, so national reference and research laboratories will continue to fulfil an important role in detecting LGV.

Serological testing remains controversial as clear cut-offs cannot be determined, and some commercial *Chlamydia* serology kits contain antigens that do not include LGV serovar sequences.

Current research aims better to understand behavioural determinants of LGV acquisition as well as apply molecular epidemiology to the outbreak. The major L2 serovar causing the ongoing European outbreaks was recently shown to be identical to strains isolated from MSM patients in western USA in the early 1980s, where the proctitis syndrome was well recognized and interestingly coincident with the explosion of (then undiagnosed) MSM-related HIV infection.

Restriction-fragment length polymorphism PCR analysis and sequencing of the outer membrane 1 gene (*omp1*) allows putative sexual network links to be established, as in other infectious outbreaks. These sorts of techniques applied to recent MSM outbreaks of acute hepatitis C and HIV infection in major urban centres have reported tight case clustering. A recently established Medical Research Council–funded study (LGV-net) aims to use these techniques, as well as qualitative interviews and patient self-completion computer questionnaires, to better define the UK outbreak, and ultimately inform effective prevention measures.

Conclusion

Sexually transmitted infections have increased in recent years, especially among groups at risk such as MSM. Molecular testing for STIs has transformed diagnostics and plays a key role in epidemiologic investigation. Certain infections, such as syphilis, HIV and sexually acquired LGV-proctitis, can mimic other systemic illnesses. Empirical treatment for LGV should be started in symptomatic rectal *Chlamydia* infection. Co-infections with HIV, syphilis and hepatitis C are common. Taking a clear, accurate sexual history is an essential skill for all practitioners. It is especially important to offer and promote HIV testing if risk is disclosed or the illness is possibly related to HIV.

Further Reading

British Association for Sexual Health and HIV. BHIVA/BASHH/BIS UK national guidelines for HIV testing 2008. Avaliable at: http://www.bashh.org/documents/1838 (accessed 12 08 11).

Chen CY, Chi KH, Alexander S, Ison CA, Ballard RC. A real-time quadriplex PCR assay for the diagnosis of rectal lymphogranuloma venereum and non-lymphogranuloma venereum *Chlamydia trachomatis* infections. *Sex Transm Infect* 2008; **84**: 273–6.

Collins L, White JA, Bradbeer C. Lymphogranuloma venereum. *BMJ* 2006; **332**: 66.

Davis BT, Thiim M, Zukerberg LR. Case records of the Massachusetts General Hospital. Case 2-2006. A 31-year-old, HIV-positive man with rectal pain. *N Engl J Med* 2006; **354**: 284–9.

Götz HM, van Doornum G, Niesters HG, den Hollander JG, Thio HB, de Zwart O. A cluster of acute hepatitis C virus infection among men who have sex with men – results from contact tracing and public health implications. *AIDS* 2005; **19**: 969–74.

Hamlyn E, Taylor C. Sexually transmitted proctitis. *Postgrad Med J* 2006; **82**: 733–6.

Herring A, Richens J, LGV Incident Group, Health Protection Agency. Lymphogranuloma venereum (LGV). In: Ross J, Ison C, Carder C, Lewis D, Mercey D, Young H. *Sexually transmitted infections: UK national screening and testing guidelines*. London: British Association for Sexual Health and HIV (BASHH), 2006; 57–62. Available at: http://www.bashh.org/documents/59/59.pdf (accessed 12 08 11).

Nieuwenhuis RF, Ossewaarde JM, Götz HM *et al*. Resurgence of lymphogranuloma venereum in Western Europe: an outbreak of *Chlamydia trachomatis* serovar L2 proctitis in The Netherlands among men who have sex with men. *Clin Infect Dis* 2004; **39**: 996–1003.

Quinn TC, Goodell SE, Mkrtichian E *et al*. *Chlamydia trachomatis* proctitis. *N Engl J Med* 1981; **305**: 195–200.

Schachter J, Moncada J. Lymphogranuloma venereum: how to turn an endemic disease into an outbreak of a new disease? Start looking. *Sex Transm Dis* 2005; **32**: 331–2.

Schachter J, Moncada J, Liska S, Shayevich C, Klausner J . Nucleic acid amplification tests in the diagnosis of chlamydial and gonococcal infections of the oropharynx and rectum in men who have sex with men. *Sex Transm Dis* 2008; **35**: 637–42.

Ward H, Martin I, Macdonald N *et al*. Lymphogranuloma venereum in the United Kingdom. *Clin Infect Dis* 2007; **44**: 26–32.

Williams D, Churchill D. Ulcerative proctitis in men who have sex with men: an emerging outbreak. *BMJ* 2006; **332**: 99–100.

16 HIV and Syphilis in Pregnancy

Nneka Nwokolo

Case History

A 35-year-old Ethiopian woman was referred from the antenatal clinic with the following results from her booking blood tests: human immunodeficiency virus type 1 (HIV-1) antibody-positive, venereal disease research laboratory (VDRL) test 1:64, syphilis immunoglobulin G/immunoglobulin M positive, *Treponema pallidum* particle agglutination (TPPA) positive. She was 20 weeks pregnant with her fourth child. She had two daughters aged 12 and 9 years, and a son aged 4 years. Her husband frequently travelled to various African countries on business.

She reported having had a generalized skin rash about three weeks ago, but had been otherwise well. Her children were born in the UK and were well. She thought that she had been tested for HIV and syphilis in her last pregnancy and that the results were negative.

What are the recommendations for syphilis and HIV testing in pregnancy?

What measures are necessary to reduce the risk of transmission of HIV and syphilis to the baby?

Can an HIV-positive woman anticipate a normal vaginal delivery?

Are there any other infections that should be considered in a woman diagnosed with syphilis or HIV in pregnancy?

Background

Maternal infection with both syphilis and HIV is associated with considerable perinatal morbidity and mortality. A study from Malawi demonstrated an increased risk of HIV transmission to the newborns of mothers with syphilis; there are, however, few conclusive data showing a clear association between maternal HIV infection and an increased risk of syphilis transmission.

Syphilis

Syphilis may result in spontaneous abortion in the second and early third trimesters and in stillbirth and congenital infection in late pregnancy. The majority of foetal infections occur as a result of transmission *in utero* rather than at the time of delivery, with the risk of infection being directly related to the stage of maternal disease. Fiumara *et al.* showed that 50% of pregnancies in women with primary and secondary syphilis ended in a pre-term delivery and 50% in a congenitally infected baby, while in latent disease 9% of deliveries resulted in a pre-term infant and 10% in a congenitally infected child.

Congenital syphilis results in intrauterine growth retardation as well as early and late phases of disease after the child is born. Early disease typically manifests within the first two years of life and may include hydrops foetalis, rhinitis, pneumonitis, skin lesions, hepatosplenomegaly and bony involvement. Haematological abnormalities are frequent, with anaemia, leukopenia (or leukocytosis) and thrombocytopenia being common findings. Central nervous system disease may result in meningo-encephalitis, obstructive hydrocephalus, epilepsy and impaired intellectual development. Chorioretinitis, glaucoma and uveitis are also features of early congenital syphilis. Many infants are asymptomatic at birth, but two-thirds will usually have symptoms by eight weeks and nearly all by three months of age.

Late disease usually becomes manifest around puberty and leads to abnormalities in the skull, long bones, joints and nasal cartilage. Interstitial keratitis, deafness and neurosyphilis are also described.

HIV infection

Although pregnancy does not have an adverse effect on HIV progression, the reverse is not the case. Untreated infection is associated with spontaneous abortion, pre-term delivery, intrauterine growth retardation and significant rates of infant morbidity and mortality. Untreated HIV infection in pregnancy also results in transmission rates of up to 30%, and although the majority of transmissions occur during labour, infection may also occur *in utero* and afterwards from breast-feeding.

Risk of perinatal transmission is affected by stage and duration of maternal disease, duration of rupture of membranes, presence of genital infections, access to antiretroviral therapy and elective Caesarean section, and infant feeding methods.

Infected infants may present early with hepatosplenomegaly, anaemia, failure to thrive, neurological disease and developmental delay. They may also present with opportunistic infections. Some children may be asymptomatic, only developing symptoms years after infection.

Management of HIV and syphilis in pregnancy

An algorithm for the management of women presenting with HIV in pregnancy is shown in Figure 16.1. Routine antenatal screening for syphilis is well established throughout the UK and since 2001 uptake of HIV testing has steadily increased, with 95% of infected women diagnosed before delivery in 2005.

Mother-to-child transmission of both infections can be significantly reduced by identification and treatment of infected pregnant women in the antenatal period. Testing is recommended in the first trimester, with further testing in the third trimester of women at continuing high risk of infection being advocated by many.

The case above describes a woman who is likely to have caught both syphilis and HIV from her husband whose job takes him to areas with a high prevalence of both infections. Her syphilis serology (VDRL test result of 1:64) indicates early disease and the history of a rash three weeks previously would fit with secondary syphilis. It is important to remember, however, that the rash caused by primary HIV infection is indistinguishable from that of syphilis and both may be associated with systemic illness. She should be examined

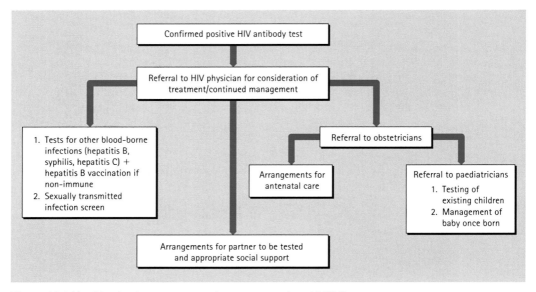

Figure 16.1 Algorithm for the management of women presenting with HIV in pregnancy.

carefully for other clinical features of syphilis and HIV infection and for evidence of a resolving primary chancre. HIV seroconversion in pregnancy carries a high risk of vertical transmission.

Further investigation should include assessment of serum biochemical and haematological parameters including CD4 lymphocyte count and percentage, viral load estimation and acute serology to exclude other causes of a rash. Her HIV and syphilis tests should be repeated to confirm these diagnoses. She should be offered a full screen for sexually transmitted infections including chlamydia and gonorrhoea as both these infections may be transmitted to her baby during delivery. The patient should be tested for, and vaccinated against, hepatitis B if non-immune and tested for hepatitis C if a risk is identified.

It is important that her husband is offered testing and treatment for both HIV and syphilis and that the patient is given adequate psychological and practical support through this process. The fact that she thinks that she tested negative for HIV in her last pregnancy suggests that her older children are not infected. However, if there is any doubt as to whether testing was actually performed, arrangements should be made with the local paediatric service for all her children to be tested, as the absence of symptoms does not exclude vertical infection even in older children.

Treatment of syphilis in pregnancy

The treatment of choice for syphilis at all stages is penicillin. The British Association for HIV and Sexual Health recommends a single dose of 2.4 MU of benzathine penicillin G for early syphilis (primary, secondary and early latent disease) and three doses a week apart for late disease. If treatment for syphilis is initiated in the third trimester of pregnancy, a second dose of benzathine penicillin should be given one week after the first. Benzathine penicillin has, however, been associated with some treatment failures in pregnancy. Alternatives to benzathine penicillin include procaine penicillin, ceftriaxone and erythromycin.

Treatment of early syphilis may be associated with the Jarisch–Herxheimer reaction, which is an acute febrile condition associated with fever, chills and myalgia. This occurs as a result of endotoxin release following sudden killing of large numbers of syphilitic treponemes. In pregnancy, this may result in foetal distress and premature labour, and consideration should be given to admission to hospital for foetal monitoring. The use of steroids may reduce the risk of this reaction.

Infants born to mothers with syphilis should be seen by the paediatricians upon delivery and carefully examined for signs of congenital syphilis. They should be managed according to standard guidelines.

Treatment of HIV in pregnancy

The ACTG 076 study showed a reduction in transmission from 29% to 7.9% in women who received oral zidovudine (AZT) from the second trimester of pregnancy, intravenous zidovudine in labour and whose babies received zidovudine for six weeks after delivery. Following this, several studies have demonstrated further reductions in transmission (to less than 2%) as a result of interventions involving various combination antiretroviral regimens (usually including zidovudine), elective Caesarean section (or vaginal delivery in women with an undetectable viral load) and avoidance of breast-feeding. Most studies also involved treatment of the infant for a variable time period after birth.

The choice of antiretroviral regimen and timing of treatment depend on whether the mother needs treatment for herself or whether treatment is to be given solely to prevent transmission to her baby. This decision is generally made on the basis of maternal CD4 lymphocyte count and stage of pregnancy. The 2008 British HIV Association (BHIVA) guidelines for the management of HIV in pregnancy advise that women who do not require immediate treatment (e.g. who have CD4 lymphocyte counts $>350 \times 10^6/l$) should start treatment in the second trimester (ideally by 28 weeks) with a standard boosted protease inhibitor-based regimen. This should continue until after delivery, at which time treatment may be stopped as long as the viral load is undetectable. Women needing to start treatment should do so and continue treatment following delivery. It is recommended that zidovudine be included in the regimen unless contraindicated. Women who achieve an undetectable viral load by 36 weeks may anticipate a vaginal delivery and do not need intravenous zidovudine as directed by previous guidelines. Those who elect to have a planned Caesarean section should be delivered at 39 weeks. The BHIVA guidelines allow for modifications to the above regimens according to a woman's individual circumstances. Women who conceive on highly active antiretroviral therapy (HAART) should continue their treatment. Most antiretroviral agents apart from didanosine and efavirenz appear to be safe in pregnancy. The association of efavirenz with foetal neurological abnormalities is difficult to establish as it is based on a small number of case reports with significant reporting bias.

Recent Developments

Studies are underway to ascertain the safety of breast-feeding by women on HAART. Until the results are known, the recommendation remains that HIV-positive women should not breast-feed. There are also ongoing studies into the effects of maternal anti-retroviral therapy on uninfected infants.

Conclusion

Syphilis and HIV diagnosis during pregnancy presents significant challenges to the HIV specialist and obstetrician. Syphilis should be managed as per the stage of infection (with benzathine penicillin) and HIV therapy should be commenced early if there is symptomatic maternal disease or a low CD4 lymphocyte count. In asymptomatic mothers, HIV therapy should start in the second trimester with a goal of undetectable viral load prior to delivery. Following delivery, babies should receive antiretroviral therapy for four weeks and serial HIV antibody and DNA polymerase chain reaction measurements to establish whether or not the baby is infected. Close liaison with obstetricians, midwives and paediatricians is mandatory.

Further Reading

Antiretroviral Pregnancy Registry. Available at: www.apregistry.com (accessed 13 09 11).

Connor EM, Sperling RS, Gelber R *et al*. Reduction of maternal–infant transmission of human immunodefiency virus type 1 with zidovudine treatment. *N Engl J Med* 1994; **331**: 1173–80.

De Ruiter A, Mercey D, Anderson J *et al*. British HIV Association and Children's HIV Association guidelines for the management of HIV infection in pregnant women 2008. *HIV Med* 2008; **9**: 452–502.

Donders GG, Desmyter J, Hooft P, Dewet GH. Apparent failure of one injection of benzathine penicillin G for syphilis during pregnancy in human immunodeficiency virus-seronegative African women. *Sex Transm Dis* 1997; **24**: 94–101.

Fiumara N, Fleming W, Downing JG, Good F. The incidence of prenatal syphilis at the Boston City Hospital. *N Engl J Med* 1952; **247**: 48–52.

Kingston M, French P, Goh B *et al*. UK National Guidelines on the management of syphilis 2008. *Int J STD AIDS* 2008; **19**: 729–40.

Mwapasa V, Rogerson SJ, Kwiek JJ *et al*. Maternal syphilis infection is associated with increased risk of mother-to-child transmission of HIV in Malawi. *AIDS* 2006; **20**: 1869–77.

Rouzioux C, Costagliola D, Burgard M *et al*. Estimated timing of mother-to-child human immunodeficiency virus type 1 (HIV-1) transmission by use of a Markov model. The HIV Infection in Newborns French Collaborative Study Group. *Am J Epidemiol* 1995; **142**: 1330–7.

Tookey P *et al*. Obstetric and paediatric HIV surveillance data from the UK and Ireland. Health Protection Agency, 2007. Available at: http://www.hpa.org.uk/web/HPAwebFile/HPAweb_C/1194947410417#2 (accessed 13 09 11).

17 Group B *Streptococcus* Infection in Pregnancy

Sophie Beal

Case History

A 30-year-old woman was admitted in her second pregnancy at 28 weeks gestation with confirmed rupture of membranes. She had previously delivered a stillborn baby at 30 weeks; group B *Streptococcus* (GBS) infection was implicated. She was allergic to penicillin.

What are the risks for this woman and her baby?

How can vertical transmission of GBS be interrupted?

How should antenatal management of pre-term premature rupture of membranes (PPROM) be affected by risk factors for neonatal GBS infection?

How should this woman's management be altered to reflect her penicillin allergy?

What treatment should be given to the baby?

Background

Delivery should be timed carefully in PPROM in order to balance the risk of chorioamnionitis and maternal and neonatal infections against prematurity. Pregnancy should ideally be prolonged until 34 weeks gestation, but infection increases with duration of rupture.

Women with PPROM should undergo frequent clinical assessment including maternal pulse and temperature, liquor colour, fetal movements, cardiotocograph, leukocyte count and C-reactive protein. There are no conclusive data to support repeated vaginal swabbing. Selected women can eventually be managed as outpatients if stable.

A ten-day course of oral erythromycin is recommended. This reduces the risk of chorioamnionitis and neonatal infection, as well as helping to prolong pregnancy, but it does not affect perinatal mortality. Corticosteroids should be given to promote surfactant production.

GBS can be isolated from the vagina of 15%–40% of pregnant women. Vertical transmission occurs during delivery in 50%. Most infants remain asymptomatic, but 1%–2% develop life-threatening clinical infection (usually pneumonia, meningitis and/or septicaemia). GBS has also been implicated in mid-trimester miscarriage and PPROM and is associated with maternal endometritis and wound and urinary tract infections.

Vertical transmission is more likely if there is heavy maternal colonization, GBS bacteriuria, ruptured membranes, pre-term delivery or intrapartum pyrexia. It is successfully interrupted by intrapartum intravenous antibiotic prophylaxis (IAP). Potential benefits should be balanced against cost, medicalization of labour, anaphylaxis risk, development of antibiotic resistance and possible increases in non-GBS neonatal infection.

Ampicillin has been used in most clinical studies of IAP, but many authorities prefer benzylpenicillin due to its favourable pharmacokinetics and narrow spectrum of activity. These features should theoretically reduce the proliferation of non-GBS and antibiotic-resistant microorganisms.

Until the production of the 2003 Royal College of Obstetricians and Gynaecologists (RCOG) guidelines, there was no UK consensus on selection of women for IAP. A risk-factor approach is now recommended, in that IAP should be offered to mothers who have had a baby previously with GBS infection or are found to have GBS bacteriuria during pregnancy, and considered for those who have other GBS risk factors (Table 17.1). The argument for IAP strengthens in the presence of two or more risk factors. Benzylpenicillin is the antibiotic of choice (3 g IV followed by 1.5 g every 4 hours until delivery). Clindamycin should be used in penicillin-allergic women (900 mg IV 8-hourly). If possible, the first dose should be given at least two hours prior to delivery.

Table 17.1 RCOG guidelines (2003) for selection of women for IAP	
Risk factor	IAP
Prematurity <37 weeks	Consider, especially if 2 or more risk factors
Prolonged rupture of membranes >18 hours	
Intrapartum pyrexia >38°C	
Incidental finding vaginal GBS	
GBS bacteriuria	Offer
Previous baby with GBS disease	Offer
GBS detected in previous pregnancy	Not indicated
GBS colonized undergoing elective Caesarean section	Not indicated

GBS prophylaxis is unnecessary in PPROM until established labour. If chorioamnionitis is suspected, broad-spectrum antibiotic therapy including an agent active against GBS should replace GBS-specific antibiotic prophylaxis.

Early-onset GBS disease is evident in 90% of infected neonates within 12 hours of birth. As any neonatal sepsis can progress rapidly to death, neonates with signs of infection should be treated immediately with broad-spectrum antibiotics providing cover against GBS and other common pathogens (Table 17.2).

Table 17.2 RCOG guidelines (2003) for neonatal management of GBS risk factors	
Neonatal assessment	Recommended management
Clinical signs of early-onset infection	Prompt treatment with broad-spectrum antibiotics including cover for GBS and other common pathogens
Sibling GBS infection	Clinical evaluation at birth, observation for at least 12 hours OR
	Blood cultures at birth; benzylpenicillin while waiting for results
Other maternal risk factors (especially 2 or more)	
Well infant, no risk factors	No investigations or antibiotics required

There is insufficient evidence for clear treatment recommendations in well neonates with risk factors. Some clinicians will commence antibiotics whilst others will advocate observation. When a sibling has previously had GBS disease, the neonate should either be clinically evaluated for at least 12 hours after birth or blood cultures should be taken and penicillin given until results are available.

Management

As this lady was initially well, the intention was to manage her conservatively as an inpatient until 34 weeks gestation. She was given prophylactic steroids and erythromycin according to RCOG guidelines.

At 32 weeks she developed pyrexia, uterine tenderness and leukocytosis. Chorioamnionitis was diagnosed, clindamycin and gentamicin were commenced and the baby was delivered by Caesarean section.

Neonatal surface swabs and blood cultures were obtained and intravenous amoxicillin and gentamicin given pending results. GBS were grown from surface swabs and blood cultures. Full courses of maternal and neonatal antibiotics were completed. Mother and baby both made a full recovery.

Recent Developments

Studies *in vitro* have shown some microbiocides to have strong activity against GBS. Chlorhexidine is cheap and may have a role in reducing GBS transmission in developing countries where antibiotics are not readily available. It has been found to have little or no impact on antibiotic resistance. Studies have shown conflicting effects on GBS infection.

GBS vaccines are currently under development. Protective immunoglobulin G GBS antibodies appear to be transferred across the placenta. Most work has focused on the covalent coupling of a protein antigen to a capsular polysaccharide. This stimulates T cells and significantly increases immunogenicity.

Recently the genomes of different GBS strains have been described, with further implications for analysis and vaccine development.

Conclusion

Neonatal GBS disease produces significant morbidity and mortality, but IAP interrupts vertical transmission. Risk-factor based RCOG guidelines have simplified patient selection for IAP and subsequent neonatal management. Antenatal management of PPROM is largely unaffected by GBS risk factors. In suspected chorioamnionitis, broad-spectrum antibiotics with anti-GBS activity should replace GBS-specific IAP.

Further Reading

Boyer KM, Gotoff SP. Prevention of early-onset neonatal group B streptococcal disease with selective intrapartum chemoprophylaxis. *New Engl J Med* 1986; **314**: 1665–9.

Edwards MS, Nizet V, Baker CJ. Group B streptococcal infections. In: Remington JS, Klein JO, Wilson CB, Baker CJ (eds). *Infectious Diseases of the Fetus and Newborn Infant*, 6th edition. Philadelphia: Elsevier Saunders, 2006; 404–64.

Gibbs RS, Schrag S, Schuchat A. Perinatal infections due to Group B streptococci. *Obstet Gynecol* 2004; **104**: 1062–76.

Kasper DL, Paoletti LC, Wessels MR *et al.* Immune response to type III group B streptococcal polysaccharide-tetanus toxoid conjugate vaccine. *J Clin Invest* 1996; **98**: 2308–14.

Maione D, Margarit I, Rinaudo CD *et al.* Identification of a universal group B *Streptococcus* vaccine by multiple genome screen. *Science* 2005; **309**: 148–50.

Pass MA, Gray BM, Khare S, Dillon HC Jr. Prospective studies of group B streptococcal infections in infants. *J Pediatr* 1979; **95**: 437–43.

Royal College of Obstetricians and Gynaecologists. Preterm prelabour rupture of membranes. Green-top Guideline No. 44. London: RCOG Press, 2006.

Royal College of Obstetricians and Gynaecologists. Prevention of early onset neonatal group B streptococcal disease. Green-top Guideline No. 36. London: RCOG Press, 2003.

Schuchat A, Deaver-Robinson K, Plikaytis BD, Zangwill KM, Mohle-Boetani J, Wenger JD. Multistate case-control study of maternal risk factors for neonatal group B streptococcal disease. *Pediatr Infect Dis J* 1994; **13**: 623–9.

Stade B, Shah V, Ohlsson A. Vaginal chlorhexidine during labour to prevent early-onset neonatal group B streptococcal infection. *Cochrane Database Syst Rev* 2004; CD003520.

CARDIOVASCULAR INFECTIONS

PROBLEM

18 Vascular Graft Infection

Stephanie J. Dancer

Case History

A 72-year-old man was referred by his general practitioner complaining of intermittent pain in the legs on exercise. He had recently given up smoking but was otherwise reasonably fit and well. Examination revealed an extensive aortic aneurysm involving the iliac bifurcation. He underwent successful grafting without complication but acquired methicillin-resistant *Staphylococcus aureus* (MRSA) at some stage on his surgical journey. Colonization soon became invasive infection and serial blood cultures repeatedly grew the organism. He was commenced on vancomycin, and then linezolid as cultures continued to grow MRSA. The surgeon was reluctant to remove the graft and both renal and liver function began to deteriorate.

How should the surgeon manage this infected vascular graft?

Why did the patient fail to respond to vancomycin?

Are there any other therapeutic options for this patient?

Background

One of the biggest threats to the success of a vascular graft is infection. This is always serious, but particularly so in the aortofemoral area. The quantity of diseased tissue found at first operation, and quality of remaining tissue, are crucial in determining the outcome of the operation and long-term survival of the graft. When atherosclerotic deposits or other pathology compromise vascular endothelium, it is difficult for the surgeon to attach the graft ends smoothly and the operative site then becomes a focus for infection.

Staphylococcus aureus is notorious for identifying damaged tissue at sites where turbulent blood flow creates an opportunity for immune evasion. Even a transient bacteraemia allows a few colony-forming units of staphylococci to adhere to exposed endothelium and set up infection. Once an abscess has formed, treatment is challenging because the organism survives inside polymorphs and non-phagocytic cells. In addition, *S. aureus* produces an enzyme called coagulase, which converts soluble fibrinogen to insoluble fibrin at the infection site, and thus creates a robust barrier to the body's natural defence mechanisms. This barrier also protects the organism against the effects of antibiotics, as does the intracellular nature of *S. aureus*.

Intravenous vancomycin is the drug of choice for MRSA deep tissue infections and bacteraemia. The dose has to be tailored according to serum levels since it is potentially nephrotoxic. Even well-managed bolus dosing or continuous infusion can compromise renal function and force the reduction of the daily dose or even termination of therapy. This is more common in the elderly. In addition, whilst vancomycin rapidly removes staphylococci from the bloodstream, it will not penetrate a staphylococcal abscess in sufficient concentration to kill the organism nor will it sterilize a graft. The antibiotic cannot kill surviving intracellular staphylococci either. Repeated dosing of vancomycin encourages so-called vancomycin-tolerant strains (minimum inhibitory concentrations ≥ 2 mg/l), which then fail to respond to therapy, so prescribing other anti-staphylococcal drugs in conjunction with vancomycin has become more common for serious MRSA infections.

What are the other drugs available for the treatment of MRSA? These include older antibiotics such as trimethoprim, fusidic acid, tetracyclines, clindamycin and rifampicin, and newer drugs such as linezolid, quinupristin-dalfopristin and daptomycin (Table 18.1). Their use depends upon antibiotic susceptibility of individual strains – UK strains are often resistant to clindamycin, for example – but it is potential adverse effects that ultimately dictate treatment choices. Fusidic acid and rifampicin are hepatotoxic, particularly in the elderly, and linezolid may suppress bone marrow function. None guarantee sterilization of an infected vascular graft. Often the only course of action is to remove and replace the graft under cover of appropriate antibiotics.

Management options

The patient concerned was elderly but in reasonably good health before he contracted MRSA. Repeated blood cultures continued to grow MRSA despite adequate serum levels of vancomycin. Renal function began to deteriorate and at this point linezolid was initiated. Whilst blood cultures rapidly became sterile, there was little change in the C-reactive protein (CRP), which remained over 100 mg/l. The patient was symptomatic, with low-grade pyrexia and declining liver function. He developed a discharging sinus in his groin, a swab of which grew the same strain of MRSA as isolated previously from blood. The organism was susceptible to all anti-staphylococcal drugs tested.

Table 18.1 Antibiotic options for hospital-acquired MRSA in adults

Parenteral	Dose	Oral (also parenteral*)	Oral Dose
Vancomycin		**Rifampicin***	
Loading required	Dependent on creatinine clearance	Always use in combination	300–600 mg 12 hourly
Serum levels mandatory		Adverse effects: hepatotoxicity	
Adverse effects unusual if closely monitored: renal and oto-toxicity	Slow bolus infusion or continuous IV infusion	May be given by IV route also if required	
Poor lung penetration	Average dose of 1000 mg 12 hourly by slow infusion		
Teicoplanin		**Doxycycline**	
Loading required	400–1000 mg daily IV or IM	Always use in combination	100–200 mg daily or 12 hourly
Serum levels may be necessary		Adverse effects: GI upset; skin rash	
Adverse effects: renal toxicity			
Daptomycin		**Sodium fusidate***	
Adverse effects: myositis, renal toxicity	6 mg kg⁻¹ once daily by 2 minute bolus	Always use in combination	250–500 mg 8 hourly
Inactivated by surfactant therefore contra-indicated in primary pulmonary infection		Adverse effects: hepatotoxicity	
Gentamicin		**Trimethoprim**	
Serum levels and renal function monitoring mandatory	Typically 80–400 mg daily IV	Always use in combination	200 mg 12 hourly
Not monotherapy	Dose adjust depending on creatinine clearance and serum concentration		
Adverse effects: renal and oto-toxicity			
Avoid prolonged therapy as toxicity is cumulative			
Tigecycline		**Linezolid***	
Avoid as primary therapy in bacteraemia due to increased mortality risk	100 mg initially, then 50 mg bd	Adverse effects: bone marrow toxicity; optic neuropathy	600 mg 12 hourly
Adverse effects: GI upset			
Quinupristin-Dalfopristin		**Pristinamycin**	
Must be given via central line	7.5 mg kg⁻¹ tds	Adverse effects: GI upset	500–1000 mg 8 hourly
Adverse effects: cardiac arrhythmias; arthralgia			
Ceftobiprole		**Co-trimoxazole***	
Adverse effects: renal toxicity; GI upset	500 mg tds by slow infusion	Adverse effects: Stevens-Johnson syndrome	960 mg 12 hourly
		Chloramphenicol*	
		Adverse effects: bone marrow toxicity	50mg kg⁻¹ in four divided doses
		Nitrofurantoin	
		Localized urinary sepsis only	50 mg 6 hourly
		Fosfomycin*	
		Urinary sepsis only	1000 mg 8 hourly

Key: GI – gastrointestinal; IM - intramuscular; IV - intravenous

NB. Use of any agent is subject to antimicrobial susceptibility testing

Please refer to British National Formulary (bnf.org) or loca/nationa/ guidelines for further information

A number of options were discussed with the surgeons:

1   Add in a small once-daily dose of gentamicin, dependent upon renal function.
2   Add in rifampicin 300–600 mg bd or fusidic acid 250–500 mg tds.
3   Stop linezolid and initiate oral therapy, using a combination of two antibiotics chosen from rifampicin, fusidic acid, trimethoprim and tetracycline.
4   Stop linezolid and start daptomycin.
5   Insert a central line and start quinupristin-dalfopristin.
6   Refer the patient for further surgery to remove the infected graft and replace it under cover of any of the above.

The surgeons chose option 2 and rifampicin was added to linezolid before a rapid increase in liver transaminases forced an abrupt withdrawal. The patient was duly returned to theatre for removal and replacement of the graft under vancomycin cover. Repeat blood cultures again grew MRSA less than a week after surgery. It was clear that there could be no further surgical intervention. Daptomycin (6 mg/kg/day) was initiated with little effect, although this may have been due to the fact that several doses were omitted due to poor intravenous access. He was given a central line, which then became infected with Enterococcus (faecal-type *Streptococcus*) and *Candida* (yeast) and had to be removed. Eventually the patient was prescribed pristinamycin 1 g tds, an unlicensed oral streptogramin, in combination with doxycycline 100 mg once daily on a compassionate basis. His CRP dropped to <10 mg/l during the six-week course and the groin sinus healed. There were no adverse effects. One year later he was still colonized with the same strain of MRSA in his nose despite repeated attempts to clear carriage, but was coping well with life at home.

Recent Developments

There are drugs in the pharmaceutical pipeline which may well have increased bactericidal activity against MRSA, with fewer adverse effects. In addition, the contents of the antimicrobial armoury are being re-examined to look for antibiotics that could be reinstituted as potential candidates for treating MRSA. Pristinamycin has been available for many years, but has only recently been recognized as a potential agent for MRSA. It is unlicensed but the intravenous form is available as quinupristin-dalfopristin. The latter can only be given through a central line. Fosfomycin is another 'golden oldie' being re-examined for activity against MRSA.

From the surgeon's point of view, new synthetic materials, some impregnated with antimicrobial substances, may replace the Dacron polymer commonly used at present. It is possible that there will be surgical techniques introduced that will allow more vascular replacement procedures to be carried out without extensive incision. These would reduce the risk of infection.

Conclusion

It is apparent that inadequate hygiene in today's hospitals will compromise the skill of the surgeon for many procedures, not just vascular grafting. The technical demands of replacing damaged vessels mean that the surgeon may only have one chance at alleviating symptoms. Graft infection in these circumstances offers little hope for a full recovery. Without the use of an unlicensed drug given on a compassionate basis, this patient would not have survived. In particular, MRSA graft infections, along with endocarditis and other deep infections, illustrate our continued vulnerability to antibiotic-resistant organisms in the twenty-first century.

Further Reading

Dancer SJ, Robb A, Crawford A, Morrison D. Oral streptogramins in the management of patients with methicillin-resistant *Staphylococcus aureus* (MRSA) infections. *J Antimicrob Chemother* 2003; **51**: 731–5.

Dancer SJ. The effect of antibiotics on methicillin-resistant *Staphylococcus aureus*. *J Antimicrob Chemother* 2008; **61**: 246–53.

Edmiston CE Jr, Goheen MP, Seabrook GR *et al*. Impact of selective antimicrobial agents on staphylococcal adherence to biomedical devices. *Am J Surg* 2006; **192**: 344–54.

Hayden MK, Rezai K, Hayes RA, Lolans K, Quinn JP, Weinstein RA. Development of daptomycin resistance in vivo in methicillin-resistant *Staphylococcus aureus*. *J Clin Microbiol* 2005; **43**: 5285–7.

Sakaguchi H, Marui A, Hirose K *et al*. Less invasive and highly effective method for preventing methicillin-resistant *Staphylococcus aureus* graft infection by local sustained release of vancomycin. *J Thorac Cardiovasc Surg* 2008; **135**: 25–31.

PROBLEM

19 MRSA Endocarditis

Christopher D. Pfeiffer, Vance Fowler

Case History

A 64-year-old female presented with three weeks of progressive dyspnoea, nausea and vomiting. Significant past medical history included cardiac surgery in 2004 with a post-operative course complicated by infection with methicillin-resistant *Staphylococcus aureus* (MRSA) bacteraemia. She had received eight weeks of vancomycin and had been doing well off antibiotics since that time. Pertinent findings on physical examination included a temperature of 37.9°C; pulse 104 beats/min; blood pressure 60/20 mmHg; a III/VI holosystolic murmur at the apex radiating to the axilla; absence of cellulitis or abscess; and the presence of peripheral emboli on the left fifth finger and right great toe. Initial diagnosis was bacterial endocarditis and she was referred for further tests and appropriate clinical management.

What diagnostic test has been shown to have the greatest sensitivity for infective endocarditis?

What is the recommendation from the American Heart Association endocarditis guidelines regarding the addition of gentamicin to therapy for MRSA endocarditis?

What are alternative treatment options for patients infected with MRSA who are intolerant of or who have failed to respond to vancomycin?

Background

Staphylococcus aureus has become a leading cause of bacteraemia and infective endocarditis (IE). The overall prevalence of IE in patients with *S. aureus* bacteraemia is around 12%. In a prospectively evaluated cohort of patients with definite endocarditis from 39 different countries, *S. aureus* was the most common organism isolated, comprising 558 of the 1779 cases (31.4%). MRSA accounted for 153 (27.4%) of those infections, and in a multivariate model was independently associated with persistent bacteraemia, chronic immunosuppression, healthcare-associated infection, presumed intravascular source and diabetes mellitus. With the recent emergence of community-acquired MRSA, one would only expect this percentage to increase.

The most sensitive diagnostic test for IE is trans-oesophageal echocardiogram (TOE), which was first demonstrated in a prospective study of 103 patients with staphylococcal bacteraemia who underwent both trans-thoracic echocardiogram (TTE) and TOE (Fowler *et al.*, 1997). Twenty-six cases of IE were diagnosed, all of which had vegetations visualized on TOE but only seven of which were seen on TTE. The sensitivity of TOE and TTE was 100% and 32%, respectively, a finding that has also been validated by other investigators.

Treatment guidelines endorsed by the Infectious Diseases Society of America and published by the American Heart Association for the management of IE recommend, for MRSA in the absence of prosthetic material, vancomycin with the optional addition of 3–5 days of gentamicin. The recommendation for gentamicin is derived from a randomized controlled trial of nafcillin monotherapy versus a combination of nafcillin plus gentamicin for methicillin-susceptible *S. aureus* (MSSA) endocarditis in which the addition of gentamicin to nafcillin decreased the duration of bacteraemia by about one day but did not affect mortality (Korzeniowski and Sande, 1982). Subsequent to publication of these guidelines, a large, prospective, randomized, multicentre study evaluating a new agent, daptomycin, versus comparator (anti-staphylococcal penicillin or vancomycin) for staphylococcal bacteraemia was published (Fowler *et al.*, 2006). This demonstrated non-inferiority of daptomycin for both bacteraemia and right-sided endocarditis. This study also demonstrated the impact on renal function of using even short courses of gentamicin (Cosgrove *et al.*, 2009).

Management of the case

Following admission, laboratory evaluation revealed a white blood cell count of $15.7 \times 10^9/l$ with 12% bands and a creatinine of 2.9 mg/dl (baseline was normal). Chest X-ray was without focal infiltrate or pulmonary oedema, an electrocardiogram showed sinus tachycardia but no interval prolongation or heart block, and TTE demonstrated moderate to severe mitral regurgitation without vegetations. TOE revealed severe mitral regurgitation and a 7 mm mitral ring vegetation. All blood cultures grew MRSA, confirming the diagnosis of infective endocarditis.

Vancomycin was initiated but blood cultures remained positive at day seven. Gentamicin and rifampicin were added but her kidney function deteriorated and gentamicin was stopped. Blood cultures remained positive for 14 more days. Vancomycin and rifampicin were stopped in favour of daptomycin, which quickly sterilized blood cultures, and one month later she underwent mitral valve replacement while still receiving daptomycin.

Unfortunately, six days post-operatively, her blood cultures again grew MRSA, which was now 'non-susceptible' to daptomycin (minimum inhibitory concentration [MIC] 8 µg/ml) and resistant to rifampicin. Vancomycin was restarted. She then developed acute interstitial nephritis, thought to be secondary to vancomycin, and new onset of back pain with positive magnetic resonance imaging of the spine for L3–4 vertebral osteomyelitis without a drainable abscess.

Linezolid was initiated in place of vancomycin, and this medication was tolerated for one month until she experienced nausea, vomiting, severe fatigue and cytopenias, with a haematocrit of 21% and platelet count of 73×10^9/l. Linezolid was replaced with quinupristin-dalfopristin but this was terminated after one week secondary to severe arthralgia and myalgia. Intravenous trimethoprim-sulfamethoxazole (15 mg/kg/day) was started and well tolerated for a three-month course. She was then stepped down to lifelong oral trimethoprim-sulfamethoxazole and at two-year follow-up she was doing well.

Recent Developments

Optimal therapy for MRSA endocarditis for patients intolerant of vancomycin or those with vancomycin failures is unclear. One potential reason for failure is increasing MICs of MRSA, closer to the susceptibility breakpoint of vancomycin, which has been a hot topic of discussion. Better definition of the tests used and MIC breakpoint will better delineate who likely does and does not have microbiological failure.

Daptomycin is now the most common alternative for staphylococcal bacteraemia, but daptomycin MICs to MRSA should be tested routinely since resistance to this agent has been reported with not only prior daptomycin use but also prior vancomycin use. For the other available anti-MRSA antibiotics, data are either non-existent or weak for bacteraemia and endocarditis. Linezolid has had mixed results both in animal models and case reports and there are safety concerns when the duration of therapy is greater than two weeks. Tigecycline has notoriously poor bloodstream pharmacokinetics and should not be used for bacteraemia. Ceftobiprole, a new anti-MRSA active cephalosporin, has recently been approved for skin and soft tissue infections including MRSA but has not yet been tested in bacteraemia. Trimethoprim-sulfamethoxazole, which is the drug of choice for community-acquired MRSA skin abscesses, had modest efficacy but was inferior to vancomycin when used for severe MRSA infection in intravenous drug abusers in Detroit.

Telavancin, dalbavancin and oritavancin are glycopeptide derivatives under investigation as antibiotics, as are ceftaroline (another extended-spectrum cephalosporin) and iclaprim, a dihydrofolate reductase inhibitor. Of note, the initial trials are focused on skin and soft tissue infection and data on bacteraemia and/or endocarditis are not yet available.

Conclusion

The burden of invasive MRSA infection is increasing worldwide and MRSA is now the most common aetiology of endocarditis in many parts of the world. The most sensitive diagnostic test for infective endocarditis is TOE, and the drug of choice for MRSA endocarditis is vancomycin. Recently, daptomycin has shown efficacy in a large, multinational, randomized controlled trial and has become the first-line alternative. When vancomycin and daptomycin are contraindicated or fail, all remaining treatment options should be carefully assessed on an individual basis. There are additional promising drugs undergoing clinical trials for MRSA. Only by carefully considering available treatment options can the outcome for patients be optimized.

Further Reading

Baddour LM, Wilson WR, Bayer AS *et al.* Infective endocarditis: diagnosis, antimicrobial therapy, and management of complications: a statement for healthcare professionals from the Committee on Rheumatic Fever, Endocarditis, and Kawasaki Disease, Council on Cardiovascular Disease in the Young, and the Councils on Clinical Cardiology, Stroke, and Cardiovascular Surgery and Anesthesia, American Heart Association: endorsed by the Infectious Diseases Society of America. *Circulation* 2005; **111**: e394–434.

Cosgrove SE, Vigliani GA, Fowler VG Jr *et al.* Initial low-dose gentamicin for *Staphylococcus aureus* bacteremia and endocarditis is nephrotoxic. *Clin Infect Dis* 2009; **48**: 713–21.

Fowler VG Jr, Li J, Corey GR *et al.* Role of echocardiography in evaluation of patients with *Staphylococcus aureus* bacteremia: experience in 103 patients. *J Am Coll Cardiol* 1997; **30**: 1072–8.

Fowler VG Jr, Olsen MK, Corey GR *et al.* Clinical identifiers of complicated *Staphylococcus aureus* bacteremia. *Arch Int Med* 2003; **163**: 2066–72.

Fowler VG Jr, Miro JM, Hoen B *et al. Staphylococcus aureus* endocarditis: a consequence of medical progress. *JAMA* 2005; **293**: 3012–21.

Fowler VG Jr, Boucher HW, Corey GR *et al.* Daptomycin versus standard therapy for bacteremia and endocarditis caused by *Staphylococcus aureus*. *N Engl J Med* 2006; **355**: 653–65.

Habib G, Hoen B, Tornos P *et al.*; ESC Committee for Practice Guidelines. Guidelines on the prevention, diagnosis, and treatment of infective endocarditis (new version 2009): the Task Force on the Prevention, Diagnosis, and Treatment of Infective Endocarditis of the European Society of Cardiology (ESC). Endorsed by the European Society of Clinical Microbiology and Infectious Diseases (ESCMID) and the International Society of Chemotherapy (ISC) for Infection and Cancer. *Eur Heart J* 2009; **30**: 2369–413.

Korzeniowski O, Sande MA. Combination antimicrobial therapy for *Staphylococcus aureus* endocarditis in patients addicted to parenteral drugs and in nonaddicts: A prospective study. *Ann Intern Med* 1982; **97**: 496–503.

Markowitz N, Quinn EL, Saravolatz LD. Trimethoprim-sulfamethoxazole compared with vancomycin for the treatment of *Staphylococcus aureus* infection. *Ann Intern Med* 1992; **117**: 390–8.

Walsh TR, Howe RA. The prevalence and mechanisms of vancomycin resistance in *Staphylococcus aureus*. *Annu Rev Microbiol* 2002; **56**: 657–75.

CENTRAL NERVOUS SYSTEM INFECTION

PROBLEM

20 Pneumococcal Meningitis

R. Andrew Seaton

Case History

A 65-year-old lady was admitted to the emergency department having been found unconscious, febrile and incontinent of urine. No medical history was available. Examination revealed evidence of self-neglect, she was groaning, her eyes were opening to pain and she was localizing to pain. Her respiratory rate was 26 breaths/min, heart rate 110 beats/min and temperature 39°C. Right basal crepitations were audible on auscultation. Nuchal rigidity was present but there were no localizing neurological signs and Kernig's test was negative. Blood sugar was <2 mmol/l.

What is the likely diagnosis and aetiology?

What are the immediate management priorities?

What is the optimum sequence of investigations and therapy?

Which antibiotic should be used and for how long?

How and when should corticosteroids be administered?

Background

A reduced level of consciousness (LOC; in this case Glasgow Coma Scale [GCS] of 9/15) in a febrile patient should alert the examiner to consider central nervous system infection and bacterial meningitis (BM) in particular. Immediate priorities are maintenance of the airway, breathing and circulation. Hypoglycaemia may be secondary to sepsis or starvation or as a consequence of alcohol excess or diabetic therapy and may contribute to a reduced LOC. Nuchal rigidity is present in approximately 50% of patients with BM but its absence does not exclude the diagnosis. Kernig's and Brudzinski's signs are extremely insensitive. At least two clinical signs from headache, neck stiffness, confusion and fever predict BM in 95% of patients.

Streptococcus pneumoniae is the predominant cause of BM in adults accounting for 35%–50% of cases, with *Neisseria meningitidis* responsible for 10%–15% of cases, *Listeria* for 6%–13% and *Streptococcus* spp. for a further 10%–12%. Risk factors for pneumococcal meningitis include age >60 years, immunosuppression, alcohol dependency, middle ear disease and previous head trauma or surgery. Neurological complications such as cranial nerve palsies (including sensorineural deafness), long-tract motor signs and seizures are more frequent in pneumococcal disease compared to patients with meningococcal disease (29% vs 5%) and mortality is similarly increased in pneumococcal infection (30% vs 7%). In this case the patient is likely to have pneumococcal meningitis in view of her older age, reduced GCS and likely alcohol dependency. Although much rarer, listeriosis should also be considered given her age and alcohol dependency.

Delay in antibiotic therapy following hospital admission is associated with increased mortality in patients with BM. In the UK, it is recommended that patients with suspected BM or meningococcal sepsis should have pre-hospital parenteral penicillin or chloramphenicol administered, although there is no international consensus. Blood cultures should be performed promptly and are positive in approximately 50%–70% (pneumococcal) and 20%–40% (meningococcal) of cases. Lumbar puncture (LP) should be performed to confirm diagnosis, although if delayed or contraindicated, antibiotic (and corticosteroids) should be administered immediately. Computed tomography (CT) scanning does not need to be performed routinely prior to LP, particularly as it may delay antibiotic therapy. CT abnormalities are seen in about 40% of patients with suspected BM although mass effects are uncommon. Abnormalities are predicted by age >60 years, immunocompromised status, history of seizures or previous neurological disease, and reduced LOC or other central nervous system signs. These clinical factors usually reflect the underlying pneumococcal aetiology and should be used to determine which patients should undergo CT scanning prior to lumbar puncture. CT-determined contraindications to LP include evidence of cerebral oedema or mass effect. Under these circumstances LP may be considered only after discussion with a neurosurgical team (Box 20.1).

In this case, a CT scan showed meningeal enhancement with evidence of reduced attenuation in the distribution of the middle cerebral artery, compatible with a previous vascular event. No mass lesion was present and therefore LP was performed. Opening pressure was 30 cmH$_2$O and cerebrospinal fluid (CSF) analysis revealed Gram-positive diplococci, a neutrophil pleiocytosis (white cell count >1000/high-power field), protein of 4 g/l and CSF glucose of 1 mg/l (<50% of blood sugar).

Ceftriaxone, cefotaxime, amoxicillin and benzylpenicillin penetrate inflamed meninges well. At high dose, the third-generation cephalosporins (3GC) will have activity against most penicillin-resistant pneumococcal isolates. Awareness of local pneumococcal resistance patterns with reference to the patient's travel history is important when considering antibiotic choice. Current international guidance emphasizes the importance of the addition of vancomycin to the 3GC when pneumococcal meningitis is suspected. If listeriosis is also possible, and a 3GC is used, amoxicillin or ampicillin should be added as *Listeria* sp. is intrinsically resistant to cephalosporin agents. In small series, and in the presence of corticosteroids, vancomycin has been shown to adequately penetrate inflamed meninges. When penicillin resistance is strongly suspected or proven, rifampicin should also be considered.

Traditionally, parenteral therapy is used for the duration of antibiotic therapy. Therapy for as few as three days has been used in meningococcal sepsis (including meningitis) with satisfactory outcome. It is normal practice to treat meningococcal meningitis for seven days and pneumococcal meningitis for two weeks. Longer duration of therapy for pneumococcal meningitis reflects the higher complication rate, enhanced suppuration and disseminated nature of the infection. Duration of therapy should be tailored to the clinical response and associated complications. Corticosteroid use is discussed below.

Box 20.1 **Management of bacterial meningitis in adults.**

1. Pre-hospital antibiotic therapy with benzylpenicillin, ceftriaxone or chloramphenicol should be considered if BM is suspected.
2. Blood cultures should be performed in all patients with suspected BM on arrival in hospital.
3. LP should be performed promptly in the absence of contraindications (see '8').
4. Antibiotic therapy should be administered promptly following blood cultures and prior to LP if this is likely to be delayed.
5. Third-generation cephalosporins should be used and vancomycin ± rifampicin should be **added** if penicillin-resistant pneumococcus is suspected.
6. Patients older than 55 years and those with immunosuppression should receive high-dose amoxicillin ± gentamicin to empirically treat listeriosis.
7. Antibiotic therapy should be given prior to CT scanning.
8. CT scans should be performed in patients with suspected pneumococcal meningitis and in all patients >60 years, those with history of central nervous system disease or immunosuppression, and those with reduced LOC, seizures or neurological signs.
9. Dexamethasone 10 mg 6-hourly should be administered to all patients with suspected BM either prior to or at the time of antibiotic administration and should be continued for 4 days in those with suspected pneumococcal meningitis.
10. Antibiotic therapy should continue for about 7 days in meningococcal and at least 2 weeks in pneumococcal meningitis.
11. All patients with BM should have audiometry assessed following recovery.
12. Primary contacts of patients with meningococcal meningitis should receive prophylaxis with ciprofloxacin or rifampicin.

Household contacts of patients with meningococcal infection should receive prophylaxis with either ciprofloxacin (adults), rifampicin (children) or ceftriaxone (pregnancy) within 24 hours of the suspicion of this diagnosis. In special circumstances (e.g. schools and universities) more extensive public health screening and assessment may be required.

Recent Developments

In a large multicentre, European study, death and neurological sequelae were significantly reduced by the administration of 10 mg of dexamethasone 6-hourly for four days in patients with pneumococcal meningitis either prior to or soon after administration of antibiotic therapy. This improvement is not seen in adult patients with meningococcal meningitis, although this may reflect its under-representation in adult studies. In developing countries, the benefit of corticosteroids in adults with BM is less convincing, although large proportions of patients with advanced human immunodeficiency virus infection and/or unproven bacterial causes may have biased results. Current recommendations are to administer dexamethasone in patients with suspected BM and review following confirmation of the aetiology.

For patients with pneumococcal disease, corticosteroids may be prolonged beyond four days depending on the clinical presentation and degree of neurological complications; in uncomplicated meningococcal meningitis, corticosteroids are usually discontinued unless neurological signs are present. The administration of corticosteroids in conjunction with antibiotic therapy prior to hospitalization has not yet been evaluated.

Conclusion

Despite modern laboratory techniques and antibiotic availability, bacterial meningitis remains a serious infection. Speed of diagnosis is critical, as is access to molecular and antigen testing for confirmation of bacterial aetiology.

Whilst ceftriaxone covers the main causes of bacterial meningitis, it is not the drug of choice for all and frequent clinical evaluation should be employed in order to assess response. It is likely that additional antibiotic regimens will be required in the future, should antimicrobial resistance rates escalate over the next few years.

Further Reading

Aronin SI, Peduzzi P, Quagliarello VJ. Community-acquired bacterial meningitis: risk stratification for adverse clinical outcome and effect of antibiotic timing. *Ann Intern Med* 1998; **129**: 862–9

Brouwer MC, McIntyre P, de Gans J, Prasad K, van de Beek D. Corticosteroids for acute bacterial meningitis. Cochrane Database of Systematic Reviews 2010, Issue 9. Art. No.: CD004405. DOI: 10.1002/14651858.CD004405.pub3..

Chaudhuri A, Martinez-Martin P, Kennedy PG *et al*. European Federation of Neurological Societies guideline on the management of community-acquired bacterial meningitis: report of an EFNS Task Force on acute bacterial meningitis in older children and adults. *Eur J Neurol* 2008; **15**: 649–59.

Køster-Rasmussen R. Antibiotic treatment delay and outcome in acute bacterial meningitis. *J Infection* 2008; **57**: 449.

Nguyen TH, Tran TH, Thwaites G *et al*. Dexamethasone in Vietnamese adolescents and adults with bacterial meningitis. *N Engl J Med* 2007; **357**: 2431–40.

Prasad K, Singhal T, Jain N, Gupta PK. Third generation cephalosporins versus conventional antibiotics for treating acute bacterial meningitis. *Cochrane Database Syst Rev* 2004; CD001832. Available at: http:www.cochrane.org (accessed 16 03 05).

Proulx N, Fréchette D, Toye B, Chan J, Kravcik S. Delays in the administration of antibiotics are associated with mortality from adult acute bacterial meningitis. *QJM* 2005; **98**: 291–8.

Scarborough M, Gordon SB, Whitty CJM *et al*. Corticosteroids for bacterial meningitis in adults in sub-Saharan Africa. *N Engl J Med* 2007; **357**: 2441–50.

Tunkel AR, Hartman BJ, Kaplan SL *et al*. Practice guidelines for the management of bacterial meningitis. *Clin Infect Dis* 2004; **39**: 1267–84.

van de Beek D, de Gans J, McIntyre P, Prasad K. Steroids in adults with acute bacterial meningitis: a systematic review. *Lancet Infect Dis* 2004; **4**: 139–43.

21 HSV Encephalitis

Christopher Duncan

Case History

A 46-year-old female presented to the emergency department with a five-day history of headache and fever associated with progressive confusion, behavioural disturbance and drowsiness. On examination the Glasgow Coma Scale (GCS) was 12/15 and she was febrile. The left plantar response was extensor. Admission blood tests were normal. Empirical treatment with acyclovir, antibiotics and steroids was commenced. A brain computed tomography (CT) scan with contrast demonstrated abnormality of the right temporal lobe with surrounding oedema and effacement of the third ventricle suggestive of raised intracranial pressure, therefore lumbar puncture (LP) was deferred.

What factors can lead to a false–negative polymerase chain reaction (PCR) test for herpes simplex virus (HSV)?

How would you diagnose herpes simplex encephalitis (HSE) in patients with contraindications to LP?

What factors influence the outcome of HSE?

Is there a role for steroids in the management of HSE?

Background

HSE is the commonest form of sporadic fatal encephalitis worldwide. The incidence of confirmed cases of HSE in Sweden is 2.2 per million per year. HSV-1 accounts for 10%–20% of the 20 000 annual viral encephalitis cases in the USA. The vast majority of HSE in adults is due to HSV-1, although HSV-2 has also been reported in cases of severe post-adolescent encephalitis. HSE occurs throughout adulthood. Contrary to popular belief, patients with HSE are no more likely than the general population to have a history of recurrent oral HSV.

Given the severity of HSE and the availability of effective treatment, a high index of suspicion is required, particularly early in the course of the illness. Clinical features include abrupt onset of headache, fever, altered consciousness, focal and generalized seizures, and focal neurological deficits. The clinical approach to a patient with suspected HSE is summarized in Figure 21.1.

When the diagnosis of HSE is suspected, patients should be immediately commenced on intravenous acyclovir 10 mg/kg three-times daily. Acyclovir has minimal side effects

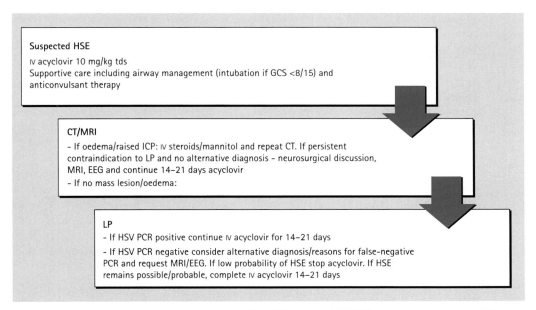

Suspected HSE

IV acyclovir 10 mg/kg tds
Supportive care including airway management (intubation if GCS <8/15) and anticonvulsant therapy

CT/MRI

- If oedema/raised ICP: IV steroids/mannitol and repeat CT. If persistent contraindication to LP and no alternative diagnosis - neurosurgical discussion, MRI, EEG and continue 14–21 days acyclovir
- If no mass lesion/oedema:

LP

- If HSV PCR positive continue IV acyclovir for 14–21 days
- If HSV PCR negative consider alternative diagnosis/reasons for false-negative PCR and request MRI/EEG. If low probability of HSE stop acyclovir. If HSE remains possible/probable, complete IV acyclovir 14–21 days

Figure 21.1 Suggested approach to the patient with suspected HSE. CT, computed tomography; EEG, electroencephalography; ICP, intracranial pressure; IV, intravenous; MRI, magnetic resonance imaging.

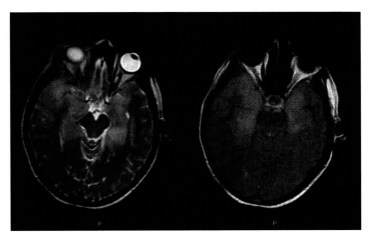

Figure 21.2 T1- and T2-weighted magnetic resonance images demonstrating characteristic appearances of HSE with focal oedematous areas in the temporal lobes and the orbital surface of the frontal lobes.

although can rarely precipitate crystalluria and acute renal failure. Supportive care for patients with HSE is vitally important and will include airway management including intubation if the GCS is <8/15. Control of seizures will require benzodiazepines and anti-convulsant therapy. Antibacterial therapy should be administered if bacterial meningitis is possible, according to national and local guidelines.

General initial investigation should be directed towards excluding simple alternative causes (such as renal or liver failure) although urgent neuroimaging is a priority. Temporal lobe abnormalities on CT or magnetic resonance imaging (MRI) are considered highly suggestive of HSE. CT is less sensitive than MRI and will be normal in approximately 50% of cases. Characteristic abnormalities on MRI include focal oedematous areas in the temporal lobes and the orbital surface of the frontal lobes which may enhance with gadolinium (Figure 21.2). If imaging demonstrates evidence of significant oedema with midline shift, this should be treated with mannitol and/or corticosteroids, and neurosurgical intervention may be required. In the absence of such contraindications, however, LP should be performed.

A lymphocytic pleiocytosis (10–200 cells/mm^3) with elevated protein (0.6–6 g/l) and normal glucose is supportive of HSE, although cerebrospinal fluid (CSF) can be normal early in the course of the disease. HSV PCR is highly sensitive (95%–98%) and specific (95%) for HSE, and should be considered the gold standard test. Even in a patient with a high pre-test probability of HSE (e.g. abnormal imaging, seizures, abnormal CSF) a negative PCR reduces the likelihood of HSE to approximately 5%, although false-negative results must be considered, and are discussed later. In a patient with low clinical probability of HSE, negative PCR reduces the likelihood of HSE to less than 1%. HSV PCR can therefore be used to guide discontinuation of acyclovir in patients with low clinical probability of HSE.

False-negative HSV PCR has been reported, and can be due to the presence of CSF inhibitors, prior treatment with acyclovir or laboratory variability. In addition, samples taken less than 24–72 hours and greater than 10–14 days following the onset of illness are more likely to be falsely negative. However, HSV does remain detectable by PCR up to seven days into treatment with acyclovir, and PCR can remain positive up to two weeks into the illness. HSV antibody testing on CSF can retrospectively confirm the diagnosis in cases where HSV PCR is negative.

When LP is contraindicated, supportive evidence for the diagnosis will come from imaging and electroencephalography. HSV serology is unhelpful in adults. Alternative causes of encephalitis should be excluded as much as possible using serological testing, with PCR for adenovirus or influenza on respiratory samples and for enteroviruses on stool specimens. Human immunodeficiency virus testing is mandatory in undiagnosed encephalitis. Brain biopsy can be performed in cases with ongoing diagnostic uncertainty or clinical deterioration, and will show mononuclear inflammation, perivascular cuffs and focal inflammatory cell infiltrates in HSE; various techniques can be used to identify HSV in biopsy specimens. The procedure is invasive, however, and may encourage intracranial haemorrhage. It is not routinely performed.

HSE remains a devastating disease, with significant morbidity and mortality even in treated individuals. Mortality rates of up to 20%–30% have been reported in those treated with acyclovir; untreated mortality approaches 70%. Approximately two-thirds of survivors will have persistent neurological abnormality. Factors associated with poor outcome from HSE are:

- Coma at presentation (GCS <6)
- Advanced age
- Delay in treatment with acyclovir
- Abnormal physiological score on admission
- Abnormalities on CT

Recent Developments

A large, multicentre, randomized controlled trial (Collaborative Antiviral Study Group 204) is addressing the question of whether prolonged duration of antiviral therapy in HSE is of benefit, and also the prognostic utility of repeat CSF analysis at 14 days, in PCR-confirmed cases of HSE. Patients are randomized to receive a standard duration of 14–21 days intravenous acyclovir followed by 90 days treatment with oral valacyclovir or placebo. All patients have repeat CSF PCR after 14 days of acyclovir. Primary outcome measures will be neurological and neurocognitive status over five years of follow-up.

A randomized clinical trial has also been initiated to investigate the use of adjunctive dexamethasone to treat HSE (Martinez-Torres *et al.*, 2008), but while these results are awaited there is not enough evidence to support routine use of dexamethasone in the treatment of HSE. As discussed above, dexamethasone may be considered if severe oedema or raised intracranial pressure is present, but this is not supported by systematic evidence (Fitch and van de Beek, 2008; Kennedy, 2005).

Conclusion

HSE remains a devastating disease and early recognition and treatment are vital. The diagnostic test of choice is CSF HSV PCR, and strategies for making the diagnosis when LP is contraindicated have been discussed. Treatment is with intravenous acyclovir 10 mg/kg tid and the recommended duration of therapy is 21 days. Randomized controlled trials will ultimately assess the role for prolonged antiviral therapy and adjunctive steroids.

Further Reading

Collaborative Antiviral Study Group – CASG 204 (DMID#98-022). Long term therapy of Herpes Simplex Encephalitis (HSE). http://medicine.uab.edu/Peds/CASG/75316/ (accessed 12 08 11).

Fitch MT, van de Beek D. Drug insight: steroids in CNS infectious diseases – new indications for an old therapy. *Nat Clin Pract Neurol* 2008; **4**: 97–104.

Hjalmarsson A, Blomqvist P, Sköldenberg B. Herpes simplex encephalitis in Sweden, 1990-2001: incidence, morbidity, and mortality. *Clin Infect Dis* 2007; **45**: 875–80.

Kennedy PG. Viral encephalitis. *J Neurol* 2005; **252**: 268–72.

Levitz RE. Herpes simplex encephalitis: a review. *Heart Lung* 1998; **27**: 209–12.

Martinez-Torres F, Menon S, Pritsch M *et al.* Protocol for German trial of acyclovir and corticosteroids in Herpes-simplex-virus-encephalitis (GACHE): a multicenter, multinational, randomized, double-blind, placebo-controlled German, Austrian and Dutch trial. *BMC Neurol* 2008; **8**: 40.

Raschilas F, Wolff M, Delatour F *et al.* Outcome of and prognostic factors for herpes simplex encephalitis in adult patients: results of a multicenter study. *Clin Infect Dis* 2002; **35**: 254–60.

Tunkel AR, Glaser CA, Bloch KC *et al.* The Management of Encephalitis: Clinical Practice Guidelines by the Infectious Diseases Society of America. *Clin Infect Dis* 2008; **47**: 303–27.

Tyler LT. Herpes Simplex virus infections of the central nervous system: encephalitis and meningitis, including Mollaret's. *Herpes* 2004; **11**(Suppl 2): 57.

Whitley RJ. Viral encephalitis. *N Engl J Med* 1990; **323**: 242–50.

PROBLEM

22 Fever and Ventriculoperitoneal Shunt

Sarah Whitehead

Case History

A previously well 51-year-old woman underwent neurosurgery for a subarachnoid haemorrhage. Recovery was complicated by hydrocephalus, necessitating insertion of an external ventricular drain. When hydrocephalus failed to resolve, a permanent ventriculoperitoneal (VP) shunt was inserted. One week later she became pyrexial with headache and diffuse abdominal tenderness. Cerebrospinal fluid (CSF) obtained from the shunt revealed an undifferentiated white cell count of 102 cells/mm³, a red cell count of 23 cells/mm³, protein 0.3 g/l and glucose 5.5 mmol/l with a simultaneous blood glucose of 7.1 mmol/l. Gram stain showed no organisms. Intravenous antibiotic therapy was commenced and subsequently *Staphylococcus epidermidis* susceptible to vancomycin was cultured from CSF. The shunt was replaced with an external ventricular drain. Three days later she had a further episode of shivering with a temperature of 38.4°C and CSF white cell count of 89 cells/mm³, again with no organisms seen on Gram stain. The following day there was no growth on the agar plates, but a nutrient broth inoculated with CSF became cloudy. *Staphylococcus epidermidis* susceptible to vancomycin was again isolated and intrathecal vancomycin 20 mg once daily was commenced. After ten days of this regimen she was symptom free and antibiotic therapy was stopped.

What are the possible infective complications of a VP shunt?

What is the most likely diagnosis?

When should removal of the shunt be considered?

Background

Ventricular shunts are mechanical devices used to divert CSF from the ventricles to other low-pressure body cavities. VP shunts are the most commonly inserted extraventricular shunts. Shunt complications include infection, obstruction and overdrainage which may cause headaches and potentially subdural haematomas. Infective complications include wound infections, shunt-related ventriculitis, bacterial peritonitis and brain abscess. Post-insertion shunt-infection rates range from 4% to 15% and usually occur weeks to months following insertion. The commonest symptoms and signs include nausea, altered mental state and headache. Fever may be absent. Typically skin, environmental or faecal flora are cultured from CSF but bacterial causes of non-shunt-associated meningitis such as *Neisseria meningitidis*, *Streptococcus pneumoniae*, *Haemophilus influenzae* and *Listeria monocytogenes* may also occur (Table 22.1) .

Table 22.1 Organisms most frequently cultured from CSF in ventriculoperitoneal shunt infections	
Coagulase-negative staphylococci	Includes *S. epidermidis*, *S. haemolyticus* and *S. warneri*; 55%–95% *Staphylococcus aureus* (methicillin-susceptible and methicillin-resistant)
Streptococci	Includes *S. pneumoniae*, viridans streptococci, enterococci
Coliforms	Includes *Escherichia coli*, *Proteus*, *Pseudomonas*, *Serratia*, *Klebsiella*, *Acinetobacter* spp.
Propionibacteria	
Other	e.g. *Haemophilus influenzae*, *Bacillus* spp., non-tuberculous mycobacteria, *Candida* spp., *Brucella*, *Neisseria* and *Listeria* spp.

Pathophysiology

The capsular polysaccharides associated with coagulase-negative staphylococci adhere well to polymers found in plastic catheters. Bacterial proteins facilitate staphylococcal attachment to the plastic. Conglomerates of organisms and extracellular slime may form a matrix structure known as biofilm; this protects the organisms from the body's host defences and administered antibiotics. Shunt material is an ideal host for biofilm, particularly if the shunt has been in place for some time.

Diagnosis

Clinical symptoms and signs and CSF examination, ideally obtained before antibiotics have been given, are used to make the diagnosis, but definitive infection may sometimes be difficult to diagnose. A negative Gram stain and normal CSF white cell count do not exclude bacterial infection. In shunts that have been very recently inserted, cell counts (usually with a predominance of lymphocytes) are frequently marginally raised despite absence of infection. Coagulase-negative staphylococci and propionibacteria are both present in normal skin flora and can cause shunt-associated infection, so extreme care must be taken not to contaminate the CSF sample during sampling. Repeat CSF examination is important, since reculture of the same organism with the same antibiogram following extended broth culture suggests an infectious aetiology. Therapy can be titrated against falling or increasing cell counts in repeat CSF samples (Figure 22.1).

Treatment

In culture-proven or strongly suspected shunt infection, an external ventricular drain is used to replace the infected shunt. Once CSF samples become culture-negative and demonstrate a normal white cell count for 7–21 days with treatment, another shunt can be inserted. Empirical therapy should be with broad-spectrum antibiotics covering coagulase-negative staphylococci , *Staphylococcus aureus* and Gram-negative organisms including *Pseudomonas aeruginosa*. An anti-pseudomonal penicillin such as piperacillin-tazobactam or cephalosporin such as ceftazidime, plus vancomycin to cover all types of staphylococci, are generally used. Intravenously administered antibiotics which have poor penetration into the CSF, such as gentamicin, or agents potentially lowering seizure

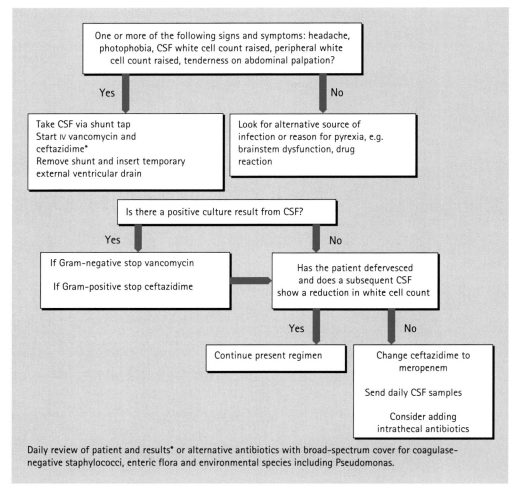

One or more of the following signs and symptoms: headache, photophobia, CSF white cell count raised, peripheral white cell count raised, tenderness on abdominal palpation?

Yes

No

Take CSF via shunt tap
Start IV vancomycin and ceftazidime*
Remove shunt and insert temporary external ventricular drain

Look for alternative source of infection or reason for pyrexia, e.g. brainstem dysfunction, drug reaction

Is there a positive culture result from CSF?

Yes

No

If Gram-negative stop vancomycin

If Gram-positive stop ceftazidime

Has the patient defervesced and does a subsequent CSF show a reduction in white cell count

Yes

No

Continue present regimen

Change ceftazidime to meropenem

Send daily CSF samples

Consider adding intrathecal antibiotics

Daily review of patient and results* or alternative antibiotics with broad-spectrum cover for coagulase-negative staphylococci, enteric flora and environmental species including Pseudomonas.

Figure 22.1 Management of fever in a patient with a ventriculoperitoneal shunt.

threshold, such as quinolones and carbapenems, should be avoided. Once an organism is cultured, the antibiotic spectrum can be narrowed to target the causative organism. Intrathecal vancomycin or gentamicin can be considered for Gram-positive or Gram-negative organisms, respectively. Several trials have assessed the efficacy of intrathecal antibiotics for the treatment of VP shunt infections using low-dose vancomycin (10–20 mg daily) or gentamicin (5–10 mg daily). Optimal treatment for this condition has not yet been established.

Recent Developments

Antibiotic-impregnated VP shunts have recently been shown to reduce shunt infections in clinical trials. Shunts impregnated with the antibiotics clindamycin and rifampicin are commonly used. These agents are active principally against Gram-positive organisms such as coagulase-negative staphylococci. There is also some limited published experience of using silver-impregnated shunts in the treatment of VP shunt infections but further data are needed before recommendation for this approach can be considered.

The role of peri-operative, prophylactic intravenous antibiotics in reducing the burden of circulating skin flora at shunt insertion has not been proven by controlled trials but is generally accepted practice. Potential drawbacks are adverse effects of antibiotics and selection of resistant organisms. Although second- and third-generation cephalosporins have been used in the past, there is a move towards agents which have a narrower spectrum of action specifically directed at skin flora. Glycopeptides such as vancomycin and teicoplanin are less likely to disrupt normal bowel flora and additionally are less likely to interact with anaesthetic agents.

Conclusion

Ventriculoperitoneal shunt infections may be caused by a range of Gram-positive and Gram-negative organisms and therefore empirical therapy should include broad-spectrum antibiotics. Successful management requires carefully timed replacement of the infected device following sterilization of CSF. Intrathecal antibiotic therapy is frequently used but its exact role is yet to be determined.

Further Reading

Albanese A, De Bonis P, Sabatino G *et al*. Antibiotic-impregnated ventriculo-peritoneal shunts in patients at high risk of infection. *Acta Neurochir* 2009; **151**: 1259–63.

Alexiou GA, Manolakos I, Prodromou N. Ventriculo-peritoneal shunt infection caused by Brucella melitensis. *Pediatr Infect Dis J* 2008; **27**: 1120.

Govender SM, Nathoo N, van Dellen JR. Evaluation of an antibiotic-impregnated shunt system for the treatment of hydrocephalus. *J Neurosurg* 2003; **99**: 831–9.

Izci Y, Secer H, Akay C, Gonul E. Initial experience with silver-impregnated polyurethane ventricular catheter for shunting of cerebrospinal fluid in patients with infected hydrocephalus. *Neurol Res* 2009; **31**: 234–7.

Lozier AP, Sciacca RR, Romagnoli MF, Connolly ES Jr. Ventriculostomy-related infections: a critical review of the literature. *Neurosurgery* 2002; **51**:170–82.

Richards H, Seeley H, Pickard JD. Do antibiotic-impregnated shunt catheters reduce shunt infection? Data from the UK Shunt Registry. *Cerebrospinal Fluid Res* 2006; **3**(Suppl 1): S55.

Stamos JK, Kaufman BA, Yogev R. Ventriculoperitoneal shunt infections with gram-negative bacteria. *Neurosurgery* 1993; **33**: 858–62.

Tunkel AR, Drake JM. Cerebrospinal fluid shunt infections. In: Mandell GL, Bennett JE, Dolin R (eds). *Principles and Practice of Infectious Diseases*, 7th edition. Philadelphia: Churchill Livingstone, 2010; 1231–6.

23 Brain Abscess

Christine Peters

Case History

A normally fit and well 31-year-old man presented to the emergency department with a severe headache of nine days duration. He had a Glasgow Coma Scale (GCS) of 15, expressive dysphasia and a mild right facial weakness, but was apyrexial and normotensive. Computed tomography (CT) scanning showed a ring enhancing cystic left frontal mass measuring $5 \times 4 \times 4.5$ cm, with extensive oedema and early herniation. His peripheral white blood cell count was $10.2 \times 10^9/l$ and C-reactive protein (CRP) was 37 mg/l. Urgent burrhole drainage was carried out and he was commenced on intravenous flucloxacillin, meropenem, metronidazole, phenytoin and dexamethasone. *Streptococcus milleri* was cultured from the pus. Five days into treatment a CT scan showed decreased ring enhancement but increased abscess size with a daughter abscess. After a second drainage procedure and four weeks of intravenous antibiotics he was discharged from hospital following improvement of dysphasia and a CRP within normal limits. Repeat CT scans demonstrated gradual resolution of the abscess on oral amoxicillin and metronidazole over four months' follow-up.

Are the CT findings specific for pyogenic abscess?

Are steroids appropriate treatment?

Is surgery always necessary?

What feature indicates a good outcome?

Background

Brain abscess accounts for approximately 1% of intracranial space-occupying lesions, and prior to antibiotic therapy prognosis was extremely poor. Despite improved early diagnosis with CT imaging, stereotactic surgery and broad-spectrum antibiotic therapy able to cross the blood–brain barrier, mortality following diagnosis of brain abscess remains high, ranging from 15% to 40%.

There are three possible routes for bacterial invasion:

1   Contiguous, from adjacent otitis media, sinusitis, dental abscess or peri-orbital infection (usually polymicrobial combinations of anaerobes and streptococcal species plus Gram-negative organisms associated with otitis media).

2   Haematogenous, characteristically forming multiple abscesses at the grey–white matter junction (usually monomicrobial, streptococci or staphylococci originating from endocarditis, congenital heart defects or pulmonary infection).
3   Direct inoculation from penetrating injury or surgical interventions (usually skin flora or environmental Gram-negative organisms).

When the nidus of cerebritis undergoes necrosis, pus collects in the brain tissue and becomes surrounded by a well-organized vascular capsule. Historically, otogenic abscess was the most common source, but post-operative and metastatic infections in the immunocompromised are now more common.

Diagnosis

At the time of presentation the classic triad of fever, headache and neurological deficit is only present in about 17% of patients. As in other neurological infections, the absence of fever does not rule out an intracerebral abscess. Diagnosis depends on CT or magnetic resonance imaging (MRI) and culture of surgically aspirated material or isolation of a typical organism from peripheral blood cultures when a haematogenous source is suspected. Typical CT findings of a ring enhanced cyst are highly sensitive but not specific, with a differential diagnosis which includes necrotic tumour, haematoma, and tuberculous or fungal abscesses. All aspirates should undergo acid-fast bacilli (AFFB) stain, tuberculosis (TB) and fungal culture, and histopathology examination.

Surgery

Urgent surgery is recommended for all abscesses >2.5 cm. Smaller lesions can be treated with medical therapy alone if the patient is operatively high risk and other sample types have provided a microbiological diagnosis. Surgical burrhole drainage resolves 90% of supratentorial abscesses with CT-guided stereotactic procedures required for deep-seated abscess. Craniotomy is reserved for multiloculated, post-operative and non-resolving abscess, while mastoidectomy is required for mastoidogenic abscess.

Antibiotics

Clinical trials of antibiotic management of brain abscess are very difficult due to the low incidence. Recommendations are based on case series and expert opinions, with no formal guidelines presently available. It is essential that antibiotics can penetrate the blood–brain barrier at concentrations above the minimum inhibitory concentration of any suspected pathogen. Lipophilic compounds such as fluoroquinolones, rifampicin, metronidazole and linezolid achieve high penetration rates at standard dosing, whereas hydrophilic compounds such as cephalosporins, carbapenems and vancomycin require higher-than-standard dosing to achieve optimum levels. Aminoglycosides have poor penetration into cerebral tissue. Ceftriaxone plus metronidazole has been widely recommended as empirical therapy (Figure 23.1). Carbapenems provide broader coverage of resistant Gram-negative organisms and excellent brain penetration. These drugs are the treatment of choice if resistant Gram-negative infections are suspected. In these circumstances meropenem is the favoured carbapenem since imipenem is associated with increased risk of seizures.

Other treatment

Steroids should only be used for life-threatening oedema, such as in this case where there was a risk of herniation. As steroids cause attenuation of the ring enhancement, measurement of abscess size is a more accurate way of monitoring progress.

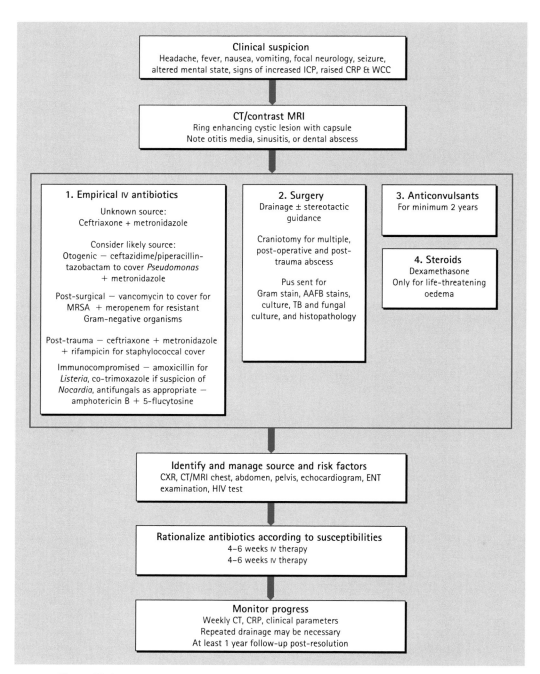

Figure 23.1 Investigation and management of brain abscess. CXR, chest X-ray; ENT, ear, nose and throat; HIV, human immunodeficiency virus; ICP, intracranial pressure; MRSA, methicillin-resistant *Staphylococcus aureus*; WCC, white blood cell count.

Anticonvulsant therapy should be commenced in all cases and given for at least two years as there is a 70% incidence of seizure.

Investigation for a primary source of infection is vital for all cases to enable comprehensive treatment. In this case, investigation included CT of chest, abdomen and pelvis, an echocardiogram, and full ear, nose and throat examination. These revealed no abnormalities, as is the case in up to 25% of patients. *Streptococcus milleri* in a frontal lobe location is highly suggestive of a sinus source. Underlying risk factors such as presence of cardiac anomalies, diabetes mellitus and human immunodeficiency virus should also be excluded.

Outcome

Repeat drainage is required in up to 45% of cases treated with aspiration and around 10% of abscesses drained via craniectomy. Duration of antibiotic therapy is dictated by a combination of clinical parameters, CRP resolution and regular CT monitoring. Poor prognosis is consistently related to lower GCS scores on admission. Neurological sequeleae can be severe, with 13% remaining in a vegetative state or completely dependent for daily living in some case series.

Recent Developments

Imaging

Diffusion-weighted MRI has been shown to have over 90% sensitivity and specificity in distinguishing abscess from necrotic tumour. MRI spectroscopy demonstrates the presence of amino acids within the contents of the cyst. Characteristic peaks are associated with specific organisms or groups of organisms. This has potential to inform empirical choices of antibiotics prior to surgery and culture.

Microbiological diagnosis

Up to 20% of samples will be negative by traditional culture techniques. New molecular technologies are being applied to improve the sensitivity of pathogen detection with interesting results. The polymerase chain reaction has the potential to give rapid identification of a wide range of pathogens, as is being applied to the diagnosis of meningitis. 16S ribosomal DNA sequencing studies have revealed that as many as 16 different bacterial species can be identified from a single abscess, as well as identifying emerging pathogens such as *Mycoplasma hominis*. Such studies raise questions about the adequacy of our understanding of the microbial intricacies of brain abscess and future work needs to delineate the clinical significance of such observations.

Conclusion

Brain abscess remains a challenging clinical entity. Prompt surgical drainage and broad-spectrum antibiotics reduce mortality. Repeated drainage is often required and follow-up is prolonged.

Further Reading

Arlotti M, Grossi P, Pea F *et al.* Consensus document on controversial issues for the treatment of infections of the central nervous system: bacterial brain abscesses. *Int J Infect Dis* 2010; **14**(Suppl 4): S79–92.

Carpenter J, Stapleton S, Holliman R. Retrospective analysis of 49 cases of brain abscess and review of the literature. *Eur J Clin Microbiol Infect Dis* 2007; **26**: 1–11.

De Louvois J, Brown E, Bayston R, Lees P, Pople I. The rational use of antibiotics in the treatment of brain abscess. *Br J Neurosurg* 2000; **14**: 525–30.

Martin-Canal G, Saavedra A, Asensi JM *et al.* Meropenem monotherapy is as effective as and safer than imipenem to treat brain abscesses. *Int J Antimicrob Agents* 2010; **35**: 301–4.

Muzumdar D, Jhawar S, Goel A. Brain abscess: an overview. *Int J Surg* 2011; **9**: 136–44.

Al Masalma M, Armougom F, Scheld WM *et al.* The expansion of the microbiological spectrum of brain abscesses with use of multiple 16S ribosomal DNA sequencing. *Clin Infect Dis* 2009; **48**: 1169–78.

Tseng JH, Tseng MY. Brain abscess in 142 patients: factors influencing outcome and mortality. *Surg Neurol* 2006; **65**: 557–62.

BONE AND JOINT INFECTION

PROBLEM

24 Diabetic Foot Infection

Paul Chadwick

Case History

A 76-year-old male non-smoker with type 2 diabetes was admitted via the podiatry department. His right foot was red and swollen and a plain X-ray showed changes consistent with osteomyelitis, with destruction of the metatarsophalangeal joint of the great toe and lucencies within the soft tissues extending across the second, third and fourth toes. There were also irregularities of the second and third metatarsal heads suggesting associated fractures (Figure 24.1). The patient was apyrexial and haemodynamically stable. Inflammatory markers were: C-reactive protein 219 mg/l (normal <10 mg/l); neutrophils 19.2×10^9/l (normal range $4–11 \times 10^9$/l). Plasma glucose was elevated at 24.6 mmol/l (normal range 3–6 mmol/l). His diabetes was managed with oral hypoglycaemic therapy, and blood sugar control was moderate with haemoglobin A1c 7.9% (normal <6%).

What microbiological investigations are indicated?

What antimicrobial therapy should be given?

What other interventions may be required?

Which specialists should be involved in the assessment and management of this patient?

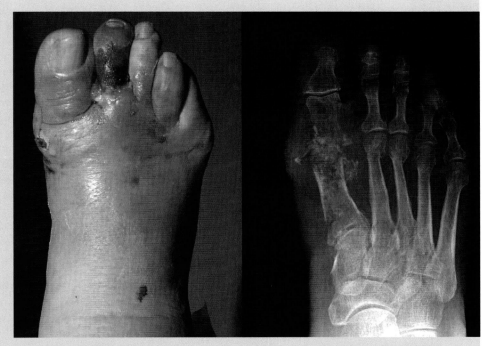

Figure 24.1 The patient presented with signs of inflammation of the right foot and X-ray changes consistent with osteomyelitis.

Background

Diabetic foot infections (DFI) are common, account for a majority of diabetes-related hospital bed-days and carry a high morbidity. The diabetic foot is at high risk of ulceration and infection due to peripheral neuropathy, peripheral vascular disease and/or metabolic abnormalities. The most common presentation is neuro-ischaemic ulceration. Good glycaemic control and appropriate foot care are important in reducing the risk of infection. Guidelines for the diagnosis and treatment of DFI underline the need for coordinated management, preferably by a multidisciplinary foot-care team including a medical microbiologist or infectious diseases physician. Appropriate wound care is essential to a good outcome and best managed by experienced podiatrists. Optimal wound care includes cleaning, debridement of callus and necrotic tissue and off-loading of pressure (including the provision of specialist footwear). Vascular surgical assessment and intervention may be required if peripheral vascular disease is an aetiological factor in the ulceration and the need for referral should form a part of the assessment for patients with DFI.

A clinical diagnosis of wound infection, based on either the presence of pus or at least two signs and symptoms of inflammation, should be followed by sending appropriate samples for culture. Tissue samples obtained from the base of an ulcer by curettage are preferred to superficial swabs and both types of specimen should be collected following cleansing and debridement. Bone biopsy with both histopathological and microbiological examination can be important in establishing a diagnosis of osteomyelitis and identifying the bacterial pathogen(s) involved. Samples should be transported without delay to the laboratory and cultured under both aerobic and anaerobic conditions.

Imaging should be considered in all patients as this can identify soft tissue abscesses or osteomyelitis. If either of these features is present, surgical intervention may be required – a surgeon with an interest in DFI is a key member of the multidisciplinary team. Underlying osteomyelitis is present in approximately one-third of infected ulcers. It is important to identify this complication since this influences the choice, dose, route and duration of antimicrobial therapy. Unfortunately, the diagnosis is challenging because of the lack of a single, non-invasive, highly sensitive and specific test. An inflamed, swollen ('sausage') toe may raise suspicion of underlying osteomyelitis. Two other clinical signs are associated with osteomyelitis in DFI: the presence of exposed bone and a positive 'probe-to-bone' test. Plain X-rays can be negative during the first 2–3 weeks of osteomyelitis and lack specificity when positive because other conditions (e.g. Charcot neuroarthropathy, gout) may produce similar appearances. A pragmatic approach to antimicrobial therapy, where osteomyelitis is suspected but plain X-rays are negative, is to treat for osteomyelitis for two weeks, then repeat the X-ray, extending the course of therapy if new changes become apparent. Magnetic resonance imaging (MRI) is the most accurate of the radiological tests available and is useful for confirming the presence of bone involvement and defining its extent. Blood tests are generally unhelpful in establishing a diagnosis of osteomyelitis, as raised inflammatory markers (leukocytosis, elevated C-reactive protein [CRP]) are often lacking. Nevertheless, a raised CRP may be helpful in distinguishing osteomyelitis from Charcot foot and, if initially raised, may be of value in monitoring the response to treatment.

DFI should be categorized as mild, moderate or severe, based on clinical and laboratory features, and assessment made as to whether an episode is life- or limb-threatening (Figure 24.2). Two key microbiological principles are, firstly, that chronic ulcers are typically polymicrobial and, secondly, that microorganisms of low virulence such as coagulase-negative staphylococci may occasionally be pathogenic, especially in ischaemic or necrotic tissue. Antimicrobial agents are prescribed empirically to cover aerobic Gram-positive cocci, especially *Staphylococcus aureus* and beta-haemolytic streptococci. In cases of moderate or severe infection, or where critical ischaemia is present, therapy can be broadened to cover obligate anaerobes and aerobic Gram-negative bacilli pending culture and susceptibility tests. Infection due to fungi is uncommon but should be considered if *Candida* spp. are isolated from a macerated wound or an ulcer that is not responding to appropriate antibiotics. Antimicrobial therapy is continued until the signs and symptoms of infection have resolved, but not necessarily until the wound has healed. Antimicrobial courses may be longer than for skin and soft tissue infections in non-diabetic patients. Mild soft tissue infections are generally treated for 1–2 weeks, extending to 3 or 4 weeks for moderate or severe disease. Osteomyelitis is treated for at least 4 weeks, typically 6 weeks, unless all affected bone is completely removed by surgery (1–2 weeks). Typical antibiotic choices and routes of administration are shown in Figure 24.2. It is important to consider a range of patient factors (e.g. age, renal function and peripheral vascular disease) when prescribing antimicrobial agents and this can be challenging. The aim is to achieve high drug concentrations at the site of infection while avoiding unwanted drug effects. Gastrointestinal intolerance of oral antibiotics, often to several

Severity of infection based on clinical assessment	Suggested empiric antibiotic choices
Mild infection Purulent or inflamed wound present • Limited to skin and superficial soft tissues • Inflammation extends <2 cm from wound • Not systemically unwell Treatment usually by oral route	First line • flucloxacillin Alternatives • clindamycin • doxycycline
Moderate infection Purulent or inflamed wound present in a patient who is systemically well and/or one of the following • inflammation extends >2 cm from wound • lymphangitis • spread beneath superficial fascia • abscess formation • necrosis or gangrene • involvement of muscle, tendon, joint or bone Treatment by oral or parenteral routes according to clinical assessment and choice of agent	Options • clindamycin + ciprofloxacin • rifampicin + levofloxacin • amoxicillin/clavulanate • ticarcillin/clavulanate • piperacillin/tazobactam • ertapenem Add one of the following if methicillin-resistant *Staphylococcus aureus* (MRSA) infection is suspected • glycopeptide • linezolid • daptomycin
Severe infection Infection in a patient with evidence of systemic inflammatory response syndrome. IV treatment, at least initially, as an inpatient	Options • clindamycin + ciprofloxacin • piperacillin/tazobactam • meropenem or imipenem/cilastatin Add one of the following if MRSA infection is suspected or infection is life/limb-threatening • glycopeptide • linezolid • daptomycin

Figure 24.2 Antibiotic selection for mild, moderate and severe diabetic foot infection.

agents, is very common and hypersensitivity reactions (typically skin rashes) are seen on a regular basis. Deterioration in renal function is also relatively common and may require modification of therapy with discontinuation of the suspected agent (e.g. ciprofloxacin or doxycycline). Good blood glucose control should be achieved as part of management of the acute infection and, indeed, afterwards to reduce the risk of future foot problems.

Recent Developments

Service developments include the provision of outpatient and home parenteral anti-microbial therapy (OHPAT), allowing patients with extensive or antibiotic-resistant infections to receive much or all of their treatment in the community setting. Research is ongoing to improve the diagnosis and management of osteomyelitis; areas of interest include the value of bone biopsy for establishing a diagnosis of infection and the role of MRI in optimizing the duration of antimicrobial therapy. Clinical trials of new anti-microbial agents are being undertaken to determine whether they are effective in treating DFI.

Conclusion

The patient described in this case history had a moderate, but limb-threatening, infection without critical ischaemia. He was treated empirically with intravenous vancomycin and piperacillin-tazobactam. The infection was polymicrobial. A Gram stain of the purulent wound discharge at presentation showed neutrophils, Gram-positive cocci and Gram-positive bacilli. Enterococci and alpha-haemolytic streptococci were isolated from dis-charged pus while at least five different species of Gram-positive cocci and Enterobacteria were cultured from superficial swabs. Coagulase-negative staphylococci were isolated from venous blood culture but this was not thought to be clinically significant. Four days after admission, a surgical procedure was performed to remove infected bone and soft tissues. *Enterococcus faecalis*, *Propionobacterium* sp. and *Escherichia coli* were isolated from deep pus and tissue samples. Seven days after admission, antimicrobial therapy was modified to oral amoxicillin and ciprofloxacin and continued for a further three weeks. A programme of ongoing wound and foot care was organized through the podiatry team as the patient had a large open foot wound post-operatively.

Further Reading

Bowler PG, Duerden BI, Armstrong DG. Wound microbiology and associated approaches to wound management. *Clin Microbiol Rev* 2001; **14**: 244–69.

Dinh MT, Abad CL, Safdar N. Diagnostic accuracy of the physical examination and imaging tests for osteomyelitis underlying diabetic foot ulcers: meta-analysis. *Clin Infect Dis* 2008; **47**: 519–27.

Grayson ML, Gibbons GW, Balogh K, Levin E, Karchmer AW. Probing to bone in infected pedal ulcers. A clinical sign of underlying osteomyelitis in diabetic patients. *JAMA* 1995; **273**: 721–3.

Heald AH, O'Halloran DJ, Richards K *et al.* Fungal infection of the diabetic foot: two distinct syndromes. *Diabet Med* 2001; **18**: 567–72.

Leese G, Nathwani D, Young M *et al.* Use of antibiotics in patients with diabetic foot disease: a concensus statement. *Diab Foot J* 2009; **12**: 1–10.

Lipsky BA, Berendt AR, Deery HG *et al.* Diagnosis and treatment of diabetic foot infections. *Clin Infect Dis* 2004; **39**: 885–910.

Lipsky BA, Itani K, Norden C. Treating foot infections in diabetic patients: a randomized, multicenter, open-label trial of linezolid versus ampicillin-sulbactam/amoxicillin-clavulanate. *Clin Infect Dis* 2004; **38**: 17–24.

Lipsky BA, Armstrong DG, Citron DM, Tice AD, Morgenstern DE, Abramson MA. Ertapenem versus piperacillin/tazobactam for diabetic foot infections (SIDESTEP): prospective, randomised, controlled, double-blinded, multicentre trial. *Lancet* 2005; **366**: 1695–703.

Lipsky BA, Stoutenburgh U. Daptomycin for treating infected diabetic foot ulcers: evidence from a randomized, controlled trial comparing daptomycin with vancomycin or semi-synthetic penicillins for complicated skin and skin-structure infections. *J Antimicrob Chemother* 2005; **55**: 240–5.

Nathwani D, Barlow GD, Ajdukiewicz K *et al.* Cost-minimization analysis and audit of antibiotic management of bone and joint infections with ambulatory teicoplanin, in-patient care or outpatient oral linezolid therapy. *J Antimicrob Chemother* 2003; **51**: 391–6.

National Institute for health and clinical excellence. Diabetic foot problems. Inpatient management of diabetic foot problems. Date of issue: March 2011. http://www.nice.org.uk/nicemedia/live/13416/53556/53556.pdf (accessed 26 10 11).

Schaper NC. Diabetic foot ulcer classification system for research purposes: a progress report on criteria for including patients in research studies. *Diabetes Metab Res Rev* 2004; **20**(Suppl 1): S90–95.

Scottish Intercollegiate Guidelines Network (SIGN). Management of diabetes. Guideline No. 116. Edinburgh: SIGN, 2001. Available at: http://www.sign.ac.uk/pdf/sign116.pdf (accessed 12 08 11).

Senneville E, Yazdanpanah Y, Cazaubiel M *et al.* Rifampicin-ofloxacin oral regimen for the treatment of mild to moderate diabetic foot osteomyelitis. *J Antimicrob Chemother* 2001; **48**: 927–30.

Senneville E, Melliez H, Beltrand E *et al.* Culture of percutaneous bone biopsy specimens for diagnosis of diabetic foot osteomyelitis: concordance with ulcer swab cultures. *Clin Infect Dis* 2006; **42**: 57–62.

Tice AD, Rehm SJ, Dalovisio JR *et al.* Practice guidelines for outpatient parenteral antimicrobial therapy. *Clin Infect Dis* 2004; **38**: 1651–72.

25 Prosthetic Joint Infection

Carolyn Hemsley

Case History

A 74-year-old lady presented to the orthopaedic surgeon with worsening pain and stiffness in her left hip. The pain was particularly bad on mobilization. The hip had been replaced three years previously for osteoarthritis and had never been as 'good' as her right, which was replaced two years before her left. There had been problems with delayed wound healing in the post-operative period. She had no systemic upset. On examination she was afebrile. She had a well-healed scar with no sinus formation. An X-ray showed periprosthetic luceny.

How can the surgeon exclude or confirm infection as the cause for prosthesis failure pre-operatively?

What is the most robust method to diagnose prosthetic joint infection here?

How much antibiotic is enough?

Background

Prosthesis failure due to infection is less common than aseptic failure but is an important diagnosis to consider because of implications for further management. With modern surgical and anaesthetic techniques, infection rates are around 0.5%–1% for elective hip or knee replacements and 4% for emergency hemiarthroplasties.

Prosthetic joint infections (PJIs) are typically classified in relation to time of onset after surgery. 'Early' infection is usually defined as the onset of signs or symptoms within three months of implantation. 'Delayed' is defined as infection causing first signs and symptoms three months to two years post surgery, and 'late' infection as the appearance of signs and symptoms more than two years after implantation. Infection is caused primarily by direct inoculation at the time of operation or by haematogenous spread.

Many organisms including skin flora, streptococci, coliforms, enterococci and rarely anaerobes, mycobacteria and fungi have been associated with PJI. This means that any organism cultured from bone, tissue and joint fluid could be significant. *Staphylococcus aureus* and coagulase-negative staphylococci, however, are still the aetiological agents at all stages. Since many of the causative organisms are those that are also recognized as normal commensal organisms on the skin, it is often impossible to decide, simply from the identity of the organism, whether it is clinically significant or a contaminant derived from the skin of the patient, the medical staff or the laboratory staff. Interpretation of culture results can therefore be extremely difficult.

PJI is associated with organisms growing in biofilm. These organisms have much greater resistance to antimicrobial killing than planktonic bacteria. The biofilms are organized structures consisting of organisms embedded in a self-produced matrix of exopolymer and saccharides. Some of the bacteria may be in a non-growing (or very slowly growing) sessile form. The pharmacodynamics of antimicrobials in the extracellular matrix is unpredictable and the matrix may also serve as protection from host immune responses.

How should the surgeon exclude or confirm infection as the cause for prosthesis failure?

No single pre-operative test achieves ideal sensitivity and specificity to diagnose PJI. Diagnosis is particularly difficult in later presentation, when chronic infection may manifest

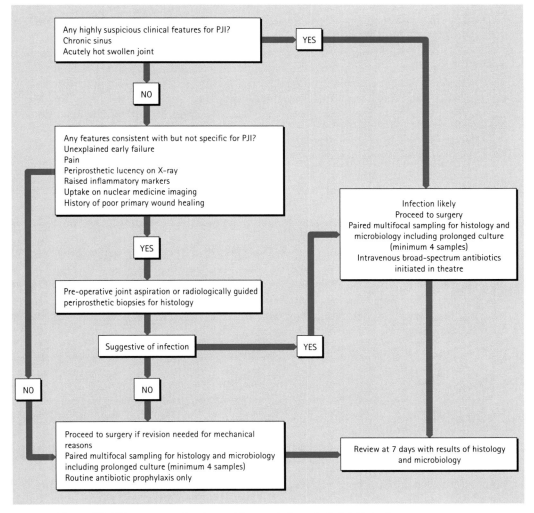

Figure 25.1 Management of patients with suspected prosthetic joint infection.

as pain and stiffness and is difficult to differentiate from mechanical pain and aseptic loosening. Pre-operative diagnosis relies on a combination of clinical history, examination, and investigations including erythrocyte sedimentation rate, C-reactive protein, imaging, microscopy and culture of joint aspirates and periprosthetic biopsies (Figure 25.1).

The presence of a sinus tract down to the prosthesis or of intra-articular pus at operation, with visible organisms on Gram-staining, are very specific for infection. Other suggestive features include a history of initial poor wound healing, raised inflammatory markers and radiographical evidence of loosening with periprosthetic lucency, although none of these are specific. Imaging artefacts limit the use of computed tomography scanning and magnetic resonance imaging. Nuclear medicine studies tend to be sensitive but have a low specificity. Attempts at joint fluid aspiration and/or periprosthetic tissue biopsy under radiological guidance are useful tests. Antibiotics must be stopped prior to sampling. Pre-operative aseptic aspiration of synovial fluid for culture has a sensitivity of 80%–90% and specificity of 94%–97% in patients without any antibiotic exposure. The sensitivity drops rapidly in those with antibiotic exposure in the preceding 2–3 weeks. A fluid leukocyte count of $>1.7 \times 10^3/l$ and a differential of $>65\%$ neutrophils had a sensitivity of 94% and specificity of 88% for infection compared to aseptic loosening in patients without underlying inflammatory joint disease (validated for prosthetic knees).

The patient underwent a joint aspiration which was sterile but showed a fluid leukocyte count of $>20 \times 10^3/l$, and implant failure due to infection was thought to be likely.

What is the most robust method of diagnosis?

The diagnosis can be made with the aid of histology and microbiology using matched samples taken at a time of surgical intervention. Sampling should occur early in the procedure after opening the joint and just prior to administration of antibiotic. Multiple samples (four to five) should be taken from different sites and with a change of instruments at each sampling. Multisite sampling is a powerful tool producing diagnostically useful information. The false-positive rate may be as high as 30% with a single culture-positive sample but this reduces to <5% with two or three culture-positive samples out of five taken (Table 25.1). Recovery of an indistinguishable organism from three out of five samples is 66% sensitive and 99.6 % specific. This methodology has been validated using primary plates and liquid culture with prolonged incubation (5–7 days). Histology showing five neutrophils per high-power field in tissue from patients without an underlying inflammatory joint supports the diagnosis of infection.

Table 25.1 Diagnostic efficiency of multisite sampling (data taken from Atkins et al., 1998)

Years prosthesis in situ	Pre-test probability of infection (%)	Post-test probability of infection (%)			
		All specimens negative	One specimen positive	Two specimens positive	At least three specimens positive
<2	40	12	33	58	99
2–4	18	4	14	32	97
4–10	8.2	2	6	16	94
>10	6.6	2	5	13	92

Given that the patient was medically fit for surgery and that her symptoms and X-ray findings suggested implant loosening, retention of the prosthesis was not appropriate. She underwent a two-stage procedure. Coagulase-negative Staphylococcus was isolated from four of five interoperative samples taken at the time of removal. The planned six weeks' intravenous glycopeptide was stopped early because of drug-induced neutropenia. She had a two-week antibiotic-free period. One of four samples from reimplantation grew a similar organism to previously and she received oral ciprofloxacin and rifampicin for six months post-operation.

Recent Developments

Detection of microbial DNA in sonication fluid from removed prosthetic material, by way of multiplex polymerase chain reaction, may improve diagnostic sensitivity over standard methods, particularly in patients who have received prior antibiotic therapy. This has the potential to better direct antimicrobial therapy. Current use is restricted to specialist centres and it is yet to translate to widespread clinical practice.

Conclusion

There is a distinct lack of data from prospective studies or randomized trials addressing the issues around type of surgery and antibiotic therapy (choice of agent, length of course and administration mode) and practice varies widely. Highest success rates (>90%) come with two-stage surgical procedures. One-stage joint replacement, debridement and prosthesis retention, or suppressive antimicrobial therapy without surgery, are alternatives. An interval of 6–10 weeks between stages is typical. Intravenous antibiotics are administered from the time of prosthesis removal and stopped two weeks prior to reimplantation. The requirement for post-reimplantation antibiotic is guided by sampling results taken at reimplantation. If specimens are clear, no further antibiotics are required. If results are suggestive of residual infection, oral antibiotics are continued for three months after hip replacement and six months after knee replacement.

Further Reading

Atkins BL, Athanasou N, Deeks JJ *et al*. Prospective evaluation of criteria for microbiological diagnosis of prosthetic-joint infection at revision arthroplasty. *J Clin Microbiol* 1998; **36**: 2932–9.

Del Pozo JL, Patel R. Infection associated with prosthetic joints. *N Engl J Med* 2009; **361**: 787–94.

Health Protection Agency. Investigation of prosthetic joint infection samples. National Standard Method BSOP 44 Issue 2. Health Protection Agency, 2008. Available at: http://hpa-standardmethods.org.uk (accessed 13 09 11).

Health Protection Agency. Third report of the mandatory surveillance of surgical site infection in orthopaedic surgery. Health Protection Agency, 2007. Available at: www.hpa.org.uk/web/HPAwebFile/HPAweb_C/1197382185219 (accessed 13 09 11).

Moran E, Masters S, Berendt AR, McLardy-Smith P, Byren I, Atkins BL. Guiding empirical antibiotic therapy in orthopaedics: The microbiology of prosthetic joint infection managed by debridement, irrigation and prosthesis retention. *J Infect* 2007; **55**: 1–7.

Stengel D, Bauwens K, Sehouli J, Ekkernkamp A, Porzsolt F. Systematic review and meta-analysis of antibiotic therapy for bone and joint infections. *Lancet Infect Dis* 2001; **1**: 175–88.

Trampuz A, Hanssen AD, Osmon DR, Mandrekar J, Steckelberg JM, Patel R. Synovial fluid leukocyte count and differential for the diagnosis of prosthetic knee infection. *Am J Med* 2004; **117**: 556–62.

Zimmerli W, Trampuz A, Ochsner P. Prosthetic-joint infections. *N Engl J Med* 2004; **351**: 1645–54.

PROBLEM

26 Vertebral Osteomyelitis

Ann Chapman

Case History

A 67-year-old man presented with a two-month history of lower back pain. He had a past history of type 2 diabetes mellitus and recurrent urinary tract infections. Three months before developing back pain, he had had surgery to resect an adenocarcinoma of the colon. On examination he was pyrexial at 37.4°C, with tenderness over the lower lumbar spine. Neurological examination of the legs was unremarkable. His magnetic resonance imaging (MRI) scan showed discitis at the level of L5/S1, with a small epidural abscess (Figure 26.1).

What are the most likely infecting organisms?

How should his infection be managed?

How should he be monitored in terms of response to therapy and the need for operative intervention?

Background

Pyogenic infections of the vertebral discs and/or bodies are uncommon but potentially catastrophic in terms of bony destruction, spinal cord damage and severe neurological sequelae. They can be acute and rapidly progressive, or more insidious, posing difficulties and delays in diagnosis. They can affect any age, although are commonest in children and the elderly. This review will focus on infections in adults only. These infections may be a primary site of infection or be preceded or accompanied by infection elsewhere. Spinal infections are becoming more common due both to improvements in diagnosis and to

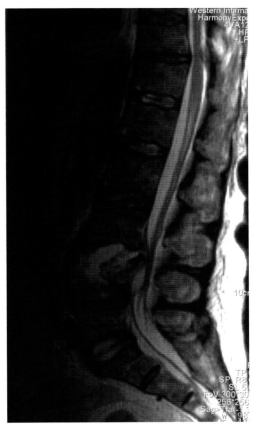

Figure 26.1 Magnetic resonance image showing vertebral osteomyelitis at the level of L5/S1. There is enhancement of the intervertebral disc and adjacent vertebral bodies, with a small collection lying posterior to L5.

increasing numbers of patients at risk, due, for example, to diabetes, renal or liver failure, drug/alcohol misuse, medical devices, malignancy or immunosuppression. Management is complicated by comorbidity, a frequent lack of microbiological information to guide antibiotic choice and lack of consensus regarding optimal therapy.

Clinical features

Over 90% of patients with pyogenic vertebral osteomyelitis present with pain which may be aggravated by percussion; the lumbar spine is most frequently involved, with thoracic spine next most common, followed by the cervical spine. About 60%–70% of patients have fever. Around a third of patients have mild neurological deficits related to nerve root compression at presentation, with more severe deficits due to compression of the spinal cord or cauda equina less common. The latter are usually caused by paraspinal collections rather than bony destruction. Inflammatory markers are elevated in over 90% of cases, although the white blood cell count is raised in only around 50%.

Patients with tuberculous discitis have a more insidious disease onset with a lower frequency of fever, raised inflammatory markers and leukocytosis, and a higher likelihood of bony deformity, paraspinal collections and neurological deficit. The thoracic spine is the most common site; involvement of multiple levels is more likely than in pyogenic infection.

The diagnosis of vertebral osteomyelitis is usually made on the basis of imaging. Plain X-rays may be normal for several weeks after symptoms develop, whereas computed tomography (CT) and MRI are more sensitive for early disease.

Microbiology

The commonest cause of vertebral osteomyelitis, both spontaneous and post-operative, is *Staphylococcus aureus*. Although usually fully susceptible, methicillin-resistant *S. aureus* (MRSA) strains should be considered if there is a history of hospital contact. Streptococci and Gram-negative organisms are seen less frequently; the latter are often associated with urinary tract or bowel sources. Coagulase-negative staphylococci can cause post-operative infections, particularly in late-presenting cases, and if prosthetic material is present. Most infections involve single isolates; mixed infections, including anaerobic organisms, are seen more commonly in the context of diabetes or immunosuppression.

Given the wide variety of microorganisms causing vertebral osteomyelitis, it is essential to make a positive microbiological diagnosis to guide antibiotic therapy – this is critical for successful treatment outcome. Blood cultures are positive in approximately 50% of spontaneous infections but are positive less frequently in post-operative infections. Culture of biopsy material or pus from an epidural abscess has a higher yield of 60%–70%, and it is recommended that patients with negative blood cultures undergo a biopsy, either radiologically or surgically, to obtain material for culture. Rarely, infections may be caused by organisms such as *Brucella*, *Bartonella*, *Coxiella* spp. or fungi, mainly Candida. Tuberculosis is a common cause of spinal infections worldwide with the diagnosis made on histology or following mycobacterial culture.

Management

The management of vertebral osteomyelitis requires a combined medical and surgical approach, with appropriate antibiotic therapy and monitoring, and surgical intervention for instability of the spine, significant compression of the cord or nerve roots, epidural abscess or severe pain not responding to medical therapy. There are, however, no prospective randomized controlled trials and there is a wide diversity of practice, although recently published treatment guidelines may help to develop broader consensus.

Antibiotic choice should be guided by the culture results (Table 26.1). If unavailable, then the regimen chosen should be based on the likely cause in that individual patient, taking into account comorbidity, possible sources of infection and risk of resistant organisms. Treatment should initially use either intravenous agents or oral agents with high oral bioavailability that are known to penetrate well into bone – for example, fluoroquinolones, rifampicin, fusidic acid or clindamycin. Current recommendations are for a total of twelve weeks of antibiotic therapy using a combination of initial intravenous therapy followed by oral agents; the timing of the switch to oral is contentious, but should be based upon improvement in symptoms and normalization of inflammatory markers. The antibiotic regimen may also be affected by presence of infection elsewhere, for example endocarditis or a localized collection.

Table 26.1 Suggested treatment options for vertebral osteomyelitis caused by specific organisms (adapted with permission from Cottle & Riordan, 2008)

Organism	First-line therapy (intravenous)	Alternative	Oral maintenance
Methicillin-susceptible *Staphylococcus aureus*	Flucloxacillin ± gentamicin	Clindamycin; ciprofloxacin + rifampicin	Same
Methicillin-resistant *Staphylococcus aureus*	Glycopeptide + rifampicin/fusidic acid	Rifampicin or fusidic acid + doxycycline/trimethoprim	Same
Enterococcus spp.	Amoxicillin + gentamicin	Glycopeptide + gentamicin	Amoxicillin
Streptococcus spp.	Amoxicillin	Clindamycin; ceftriaxone	Amoxicillin; clindamycin
Gram-negative organisms	Ceftriaxone + gentamicin/ciprofloxacin	Carbapenem + gentamicin/ciprofloxacin	Ciprofloxacin
Anaerobes	Clindamycin	Carbapenem; metronidazole	Clindamycin

In the case described here, blood cultures were negative. The patient had a history of diabetes and a wide range of pathogens was possible, including MRSA in view of his recent hospital contact, and Gram-negative/anaerobic organisms from his previous urinary infections and bowel surgery. He proceeded to a CT-guided biopsy and material from this grew the Gram-negative bacillus *Proteus mirabilis*. He was treated with intravenous ceftriaxone for twelve weeks and responded well.

Monitoring therapy

Patients should be monitored clinically for defervescence and improvements in pain and inflammatory markers. Plain radiographs are recommended at one and three months of therapy, and three months after treatment completion. Routine MRI scans during therapy are not predictive of treatment failure and may be misleading in showing radiological deterioration in parallel with clinical improvement. Clinical parameters are more useful in predicting poor outcome, and can be used to select patients at high risk of treatment failure for further targeted imaging.

Recent Developments

The increasing frequency of spinal infections (and particularly healthcare-associated infections) and the frequent need for prolonged parenteral antibiotic therapy have highlighted this patient group, along with other patients with bone and joint infection, as one which may benefit from ambulatory management via outpatient parenteral antibiotic therapy programmes. Although well established in North America this modality of therapy, which provides parenteral therapy without the need for an overnight hospital stay, is proving increasingly useful in Europe and other parts of the world in reducing length of hospitalization and improving quality of life.

Conclusion

Spinal infections are becoming increasingly common and should be considered in patients with chronic back pain, particularly where there are systemic signs of sepsis. With the increasing complexity of infections in frequently debilitated hosts, it is essential to establish a microbiological diagnosis wherever possible, so that treatment can be tailored to the infecting organism. Until recently, there was little consensus on how to manage spinal infections and only a limited research base on which to base guidelines. Current recommendations are to treat with antibiotics for twelve weeks, with clinical monitoring to allow early detection of poor outcome. Surgical intervention may be required for instability, epidural abscesses, neurological deficits or severe pain unresponsive to medical therapy.

Further Reading

Cottle L, Riordan T. Infectious spondylodiscitis. *J Infect* 2008; **56**: 401–12.

Darley ESR, MacGowan AP. Antibiotic treatment of Gram-positive bone and joint infections. *J Antimicrob Chemother* 2004; **53**: 928–35.

Friedman JA, Maher CO, Quast LM, McClelland RL, Ebersold MJ. Spontaneous disc space infections in adults. *Surg Neurol* 2002; **57**: 81–6.

Gasbarrini AL, Bertoldi E, Mazetti M *et al*. Clinical features, diagnostic and therapeutic approaches to haematogenous vertebral osteomyelitis. *Eur Rev Med Pharmacol Sci* 2005; **9**: 53–66.

Grados F, Lescure FX, Senneville E, Flipo RM, Schmit JL, Fardellone P. Suggestions for managing pyogenic (non-tuberculous) discitis in adults. *Joint Bone Spine* 2007; **74**: 133–9.

Hadjipavlou AG, Mader JT, Necessary JT, Muffoletto AJ. Hematogenous pyogenic spinal infections and their surgical management. *Spine* 2000; **25**: 1668–79.

Honan M, White GW, Eisenberg GM. Spontaneous infectious discitis in adults. *Am J Med* 1996; **100**: 85–9.

Kapeller P, Fazekas F, Krametter D *et al*. Pyogenic infectious spondylitis: clinical, laboratory and MRI features. *Eur Neurol* 1997; **38**: 94–8.

Kowalski TJ, Berbari EF, Huddleston PM, Steckelberg JM, Osmon DR. Do follow-up imaging examinations provide useful prognostic information in patients with spine infection? *Clin Infect Dis* 2006; **43**: 172–9.

Legrand E, Flipo RM, Guggenbuhl P *et al*. Management of nontuberculous infectious discitis. Treatments used in 110 patients admitted to 12 teaching hospitals in France. *Joint Bone Spine* 2001; **68**: 504–9.

Lillie P, Thaker H, Moss P *et al*. Healthcare associated discitis in the era of antimicrobial resistance. *J Clin Rheumatol* 2008; **14**: 234–7.

Mackenzie AR, Laing RB, Smith CC, Kaar GF, Smith FW. Spinal epidural abscess: the importance of early diagnosis and treatment. *J Neurol Neurosurg Psychiatry* 1998; **65**: 209–12.

Société de Pathologie Infectieuse de Langue Franaise (SPILF). Recommandations pour la practique clinique. Spondylodiscites infectieuses primitives, et secondaires à un geste intra-discal, sans mise en place de matériel. (Primary infectious spondylitis, and following intradiscal procedure, without prothesis.) *Med Mal Infect* 2007; **37**: 554–72. Available at: http://www.infectiologie.com/site/medias/_documents/consensus/2007-Spondylodiscites-Court.pdf (accessed 13 09 11).

Turgut M. Spinal tuberculosis (Pott's disease): its clinical presentation, surgical management, and outcome. A survey study on 694 patients. *Neurosurg Rev* 2001; **24**: 8–13.

Varma R, Lander P, Assaf A. Imaging of pyogenic infectious spondylodiskitis. *Radiol Clin North Am* 2001; **39**: 203–13.

27 Spontaneous Bacterial Peritonitis

Stewart Campbell

Case History

A 63-year-old woman was admitted to hospital due to abdominal swelling unresponsive to diuretic therapy. She had been diagnosed with primary biliary cirrhosis five years earlier and was asymptomatic until six months ago when abdominal and ankle swelling had developed. Diuretic therapy did not reduce the swelling and she had been placed on the liver transplant waiting list. On the day of admission she underwent large volume paracentesis but there was rapid reaccumulation of her ascites. Microscopy, culture and cell count of the fluid obtained at initial therapeutic paracentesis were normal. One week later her conscious level deteriorated. An attempt at subsequent paracentesis was unsuccessful and she did not respond to empirical treatment with a third-generation cephalosporin (ceftriaxone), lactulose and intravenous fluids. Her C-reactive protein (CRP) was 25 mg/l (normal <6 mg/l).

What is the most likely diagnosis?

Why is she failing to respond to therapy?

What additional type of therapy should be used, and why?

What is her prognosis?

Background

The deterioration in conscious level is due to hepatic encephalopathy. This is commonly precipitated by infection, dehydration, electrolyte imbalance or constipation. Spontaneous bacterial peritonitis (SBP) should always be suspected if there is any form of clinical deterioration in a patient with ascites and cirrhosis. SBP often has few or no abdominal symptoms and does not stimulate an intense inflammatory response or markedly raised CRP. Approximately one in ten cirrhotic patients has SBP on admission to hospital, and in those who develop complications the prevalence of SBP rises (e.g. approximately one in two of those with variceal haemorrhage will have SBP). Death from SBP usually occurs because of progressive renal failure, despite successful treatment of the infection with antibiotics in the majority of diagnosed cases. We now realize that ascites and renal impairment in cirrhosis have the same cause, and represent different places on the spectrum of disease severity. Hence patients with cirrhosis, who have an evolving systemic hypotension due to splanchnic vasodilatation, can be expected to progress from an asymptomatic stage onto ascites, then to diuretic-resistant ascites (now classified as type II hepatorenal syndrome), progressive renal failure (type I hepatorenal syndrome) and ultimately death, due to progressive renal artery vasoconstriction and avid renal sodium retention. The presence of infection accelerates this process, but this acceleration can be reversed by supporting the circulation if it has an acute precipitant such as SBP.

Management options

It may be tempting for a junior doctor who is faced with performing an unfamiliar, difficult or previously unsuccessful technical procedure to embark on empirical therapy rather than obtain a sample for diagnosis. In a hospital setting, clinicians should not settle for a diagnosis of SBP without either a raised ascitic fluid polymorph count or positive culture; ascitic fluid cultures will only be positive in 40% of cases, however (Figure 27.1). Even if antibiotic therapy is successful, there are implications of a diagnosis of SBP over and above the correct immediate choice of antibiotic. SBP is an indication for referral for liver transplant assessment, and for prophylactic antibiotic therapy, because the one-year recurrence and survival rates are 70% and 40%, respectively. Coagulopathy is not a contraindication to diagnostic paracentesis (and indeed a mild coagulopathy, at least, can be expected in most patients at risk).

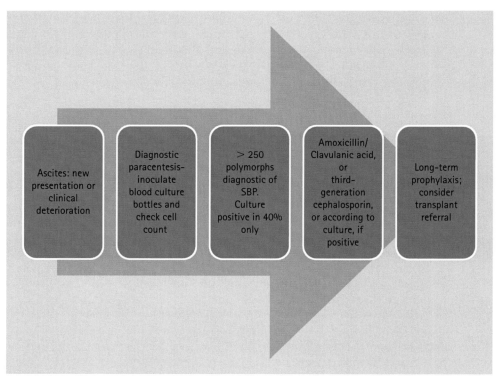

Figure 27.1 Diagnostic and management sequence for suspected SBP.

Although unlikely, if it had again proved impossible to obtain a small sample of ascitic fluid (approximately 20 ml is ideal) using ultrasound guidance then consideration should be given to alternative antibiotics, with the choice determined by both the patient's history (e.g. prior infections with resistant organisms, prior procedures, prior antibiotic prophylaxis) and the prevalence of particular resistant organisms in that hospital (Figure 27.2). In this case, the recent therapeutic paracentesis makes infection with skin-derived staphylococci or streptococci a possibility.

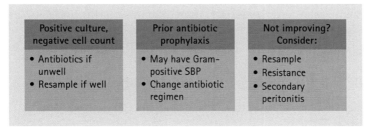

Positive culture, negative cell count	Prior antibiotic prophylaxis	Not improving? Consider:
• Antibiotics if unwell • Resample if well	• May have Gram-positive SBP • Change antibiotic regimen	• Resample • Resistance • Secondary peritonitis

Figure 27.2 Factors influencing antibiotic management decisions in suspected SBP.

Outcome

A further attempt at diagnostic paracentesis was successful using ultrasound guidance. The fluid was inoculated directly into blood culture bottles (associated with a higher yield) as well as a sterile container for cell count. There were 280 polymorphs/mm^3 in the ascitic fluid and culture grew a multiresistant extended spectrum β-lactamase (ESBL) *Klebsiella pneumoniae*. The patient received intravenous meropenem and albumin. Within 36 hours her conscious level had returned to normal. She survived this episode of sepsis, but in subsequent months developed progressive renal impairment and died whilst on the transplant waiting list.

Recent Developments

The landmark publication by Sort *et al.* advocating albumin in the management of SBP is now more than a decade old. This publication showed an absolute reduction in mortality of 19% with albumin in addition to cefotaxime. Controversy remains over the best fluid regimen to use, however, and whether use of albumin can be reserved for those with a greater degree of liver dysfunction. Most clinicians use intravenous albumin 1.5 g/kg on day one, then 1 g/kg from day three.

Long-term secondary antibiotic prophylaxis with norfloxacin following an episode of SBP reduces the SBP recurrence rate from 68% to 20%. Prophylaxis is recommended by international guidelines, with cautions regarding selection of resistant organisms.

As the protein content of ascitic fluid falls, the likelihood of developing SBP increases. Hence, primary antibiotic prophylaxis for cirrhotic patients with ascitic protein content below 15 g/l has been considered. Studies demonstrate an absolute reduction in SBP rates of 10%–20% at one year using quinolones, but the impact on mortality is less certain. In the longer term we might expect a decreased survival advantage due to emergence of antibiotic resistance in this cohort, not apparent in the original trial data, and a consensus is still lacking about the use of primary prophylaxis.

Conclusion

 Spontaneous bacterial peritonitis should be suspected in all cirrhotic patients with ascites on admission to hospital, and also if there is any clinical deterioration. Clinicians should attempt to make a definitive diagnosis wherever possible. Treatment to support the circulation (e.g. with albumin), secondary antibiotic prophylaxis and consideration for transplant referral are all important parts of the management.

Further Reading

 European Association for the Study of the Liver. EASL clinical practice guidelines on the management of ascites, spontaneous bacterial peritonitis, and hepatorenal syndrome in cirrhosis. *J Hepatol* 2010; **53**: 397–417.

Fernández J, Navasa M, Planas R *et al*. Primary prophylaxis of spontaneous bacterial peritonitis delays hepatorenal syndrome and improves survival in cirrhosis. *Gastroenterology* 2007; **133**: 818–24.

Salerno F, Gerbes A, Ginès P, Wong F, Arroyo V. Diagnosis, prevention and treatment of hepatorenal syndrome in cirrhosis. *Gut* 2007; **56**: 1310–18.

Sort P, Navasa M, Arroyo V *et al*. Effect of intravenous albumin on renal impairment and mortality in patients with cirrhosis and spontaneous bacterial peritonitis. *N Engl J Med* 1999; **341**: 403–9.

PROBLEM

28 Intra-abdominal Sepsis

Andrew Berrington

Case History

 A 32-year-old man was admitted to the intensive care unit with alcoholic pancreatitis. He was treated with cefuroxime and metronidazole and initially stabilized, but he became more unwell after a few days with deteriorating indices of sepsis. Following a computed tomography scan he underwent open pancreatic debridement from which specimens subsequently grew *Enterococcus faecium*. He improved following the procedure and some teicoplanin, but after a further week he had deteriorated again, with purulent fluid in the abdominal drains and worsening sepsis.

Why was he treated initially with cefuroxime and metronidazole?

What were the benefits and limitations of teicoplanin during the earlier deterioration?

How should the current episode be managed?

Background

Intra-abdominal sepsis has many and various causes but pancreatitis serves to illustrate some of the challenges of prolonged surgical admissions complicated by multiple episodes of infection. It is important to remember, though, that the primary pathology, inflammation of the pancreas, is usually non-infective. The most common causes of pancreatitis are gallstones, whereby stones formed in the gallbladder or bile duct migrate into the pancreatic duct and impede its drainage, and alcohol, which probably has a direct toxic effect. The process becomes self-sustaining after initiation of inflammation as pancreatic enzymes that would normally aid digestion in the gut set to work digesting the pancreas and surrounding structures. Once pancreatitis is established, infection of the damaged tissues caused by enteric organisms is a common consequence.

The role of antibiotics in pancreatitis has been debated for many years. Current consensus is that severe cases should receive antibiotics, but the initial rationale is prophylaxis rather than therapy, i.e. antibiotics are given to prevent the inflamed (but initially sterile) pancreatic tissue from becoming secondarily infected. In this particular case prophylaxis was given in the form of cefuroxime and metronidazole. It makes sense to use agents like this, that are active against enteric organisms such as coliforms and anaerobes, but there are no clinical data on which to base the choice of drug. UK guidelines which used to advise a cefuroxime/metronidazole combination now stop short from making a specific recommendation. Doctors who wish to use prophylaxis must decide for themselves whether to use traditional regimens or whether to use broad-spectrum agents or those which are known to penetrate better into inflamed pancreatic tissue. Based on limited data, many people use carbapenem agents (ertapenem, imipenem or meropenem) and some routinely add an antifungal agent such as fluconazole. Furthermore, and in common with many antibacterial strategies, the duration of treatment comes down to custom, practice and educated guesswork: 7-, 10- or 14-day courses are typical.

Despite prophylaxis, this patient's pancreas became infected with *Enterococcus faecium*. It is quite common for enterococci to emerge and cause complications in patients with abdominal problems treated with cephalosporins, since these organisms inhabit the colon (they are also known as 'faecal-type streptococci') and they are intrinsically resistant to cephalosporins. Among the enterococci, *E. faecium* is more resistant than *E. faecalis* and in particular is resistant to aminopenicillins such as amoxicillin. *E. faecium* is also resistant to carbapenems so in this case prophylaxis with meropenem would not have been any more successful. *E. faecium* is usually susceptible to glycopeptides (vancomycin and teicoplanin) although resistant strains are seen and in some countries are common. The organism is usually susceptible to linezolid, daptomycin, tigecycline and quinupristin-dalfopristin, and variably susceptible to chloramphenicol and tetracycline. None of these is without problems and the management of intra-abdominal *E. faecium* infections can be very difficult. In this case teicoplanin was chosen, although penetration of teicoplanin into abdominal tissues has not been extensively studied and by extrapolation from other data is probably limited. Linezolid and tigecycline have reasonable tissue penetration and might have been preferred, and chloramphenicol should not be forgotten as an effective agent whose potential toxicity can be justified in life-threatening infection.

The patient improved in association with surgical debridement and teicoplanin but a week later he again became unwell. The challenge now is to initiate appropriate empirical antibiotics while waiting for further microbiological information. Patients like this can spend many weeks in intensive care and often experience multiple infective episodes. It is important to make a clear diagnosis of intra-abdominal infection since the fact that the drainage has become purulent is not conclusive evidence that the abdomen is the source of his deterioration. Other possibilities include ventilator-associated pneumonia, line-related infection, catheter-related urinary tract infection, wound infection, intercurrent stroke or myocardial infarction, any of which might present with a systemic inflammatory response. If clinical evidence suggests an abdominal source (which is not unlikely given the presence of drains and inflamed tissue) then there should be an attempt at an aetiological diagnosis.

Pending culture results, antibiotics will need to be chosen on empirical grounds although the choice might be aided by Gram staining of the fluid, earlier culture results or knowledge of prevailing organisms in the hospital environment. It would be sensible in this situation to plan de-escalation therapy, i.e. to begin with broad-spectrum drugs with a view to narrowing the spectrum once the cause is established. In this case he was started on: meropenem to cover resistant Gram-negative organisms that might have emerged under cefuroxime pressure or been acquired from the intensive care unit environment; linezolid for Gram-positive cover; metronidazole for anaerobic cover (although both meropenem and linezolid are active against many anaerobes); and fluconazole due to risk of yeast superinfection in these patients. Drain-fluid specimens subsequently grew *E. faecium* again plus *Candida albicans*, but no Gram-negative bacteria, so the meropenem was stopped. He underwent further pancreatic debridement, spent two weeks on linezolid and fluconazole, and after further setbacks eventually made a good recovery.

Recent Developments

In the management of acute pancreatitis it is likely that the role of antibiotic prophylaxis will come to be better understood. Recent years have seen the publication of the first randomized controlled trials to address this and these have not found evidence to support prophylaxis; more evidence is needed but the pendulum might swing away from prophylaxis in future.

In abdominal sepsis more generally, the major drivers of change are better surgical techniques (which reduce the risk of anastomotic leakage or permit better debridement of infected tissues), improved imaging for clearer diagnosis, and incremental improvements in intensive care. The availability of newer antimicrobial drugs can be important for some patients but overall makes a relatively minor contribution to either prevention or treatment. Intra-abdominal sepsis is often polymicrobial, however, and frequently involves hospital-acquired pathogens so the spread of antibiotic resistance, despite countermeasures such as improved antibiotic stewardship, is likely to produce more and greater challenges in the future.

Common pathogens in intra-abdominal infections

Common pathogens in intra-abdominal infections are shown in Table 28.1. The term intra-abdominal infection is difficult to define. It usually excludes infections of the urological system, so perhaps 'intra-abdominal but not retroperitoneal' would be preferable; alternatively, retroperitoneal itself is a misnomer since the peritoneum is reflected forwards over the contents of the abdomen. More confusingly still, the term excludes infections of the gut lumen such as gastroenteritis and colitis, but usually includes infections of the bile and pancreatic ducts. The common theme is that normally sterile tissues become infected with bacteria that arise from within the gut, in which normal habitat they are harmless or even necessary. Intra-abdominal infections are therefore not 'caught' in the sense of being acquired and becoming infected by a new and virulent organism, but are a consequence of some other process, often involving obstruction, stasis or perforation, that allows bacteria to proliferate where they otherwise would not. Polymicrobial abscess formation is common and surgical drainage often necessary.

Table 28.1 Common pathogens in intra-abdominal infections

Informal term	Species	Comments
Coliforms	Members of the family Enterobacteriaciae, mainly *E. coli* but also *Klebsiella* spp., *Enterobacter* spp., *Proteus* spp. and others	Once reliably susceptible to cephalosporins, the spread of cephalosporinases is causing much greater reliance on other agents such as carbapenems
Enterococci, 'faecal–type streptococci'	*Enterococcus faecalis, Enterococcus faecium*	Enterococci are intrinsically resistant to cephalosporins; *E. faecalis* is usually susceptible to amoxicillin whereas *E. faecium* is usually not. In some areas glycopeptide resistance is common
'Strep. milleri'	Now known as the Streptococcus anginosus group: *Streptococcus anginosus, Streptococcus intermedius, Streptococcus constellatus*	These organisms have a propensity to form abscesses often in conjunction with anaerobes; they are usually susceptible to penicillins but antibiotics alone are unlikely to be curative unless pus is released
Anaerobes	*Clostridium* spp., *Bacteroides* spp., anaerobic streptococci, etc.	A huge, diverse and fascinating group, usually conflated by clinical microbiologists because they can be difficult to distinguish in the laboratory and because speciation is not a prerequisite for effective management

Conclusion

The goals of antimicrobial management of intra-abdominal sepsis are to minimize the risk of infection through judicious use of prophylaxis, early treatment of infection with aggressive targeting of suspected or identified pathogens, and an holistic approach that recognizes the risks as well as the benefits of antimicrobial therapy for patients who might spend many weeks at high risk of complications. As always, the most important aspect is multidisciplinary teamwork with close liaison between microbiologists, surgeons and intensive care staff.

Further Reading

Dellinger EP, Tellado JM, Soto NE *et al*. Early antibiotic treatment for severe acute necrotizing pancreatitis: a randomized, double-blind, placebo-controlled study. *Ann Surg* 2007; **245**: 674–83.

Isenmann R, Rünzi M, Kron M *et al*. Prophylactic antibiotic treatment in patients with predicted severe acute pancreatitis: a placebo-controlled, double-blind trial. *Gastroenterology* 2004; **126**: 997–1004.

Kingsnorth A, O'Reilly D. Acute pancreatitis. *BMJ* 2006; **332**: 1072–6.

Villatoro E, Bassi C, Larvin M. Antibiotic therapy for prophylaxis against infection of pancreatic necrosis in acute pancreatitis. *Cochrane Database Syst Rev* 2006; CD002941.

UK Working Party on Acute Pancreatitis. UK guidelines for the management of acute pancreatitis. *Gut* 2005; **54**: iii1–9.

PROBLEM

29 Liver Abscess

Dugal Baird

Case History

A 75-year-old woman was admitted with right upper-quadrant discomfort, weight loss and anorexia. Ultrasonography showed multiple hepatic lesions, interpreted as malignant metastases, and she was discharged home with a diagnosis of carcinomatosis. Three months later, when admitted for respite care, her temperature was noted to be 38.5°C, and blood cultures grew *Streptococcus milleri*. The microbiologist advised that the diagnosis of multiple liver abscesses should be considered. Percutaneous computed tomography (CT)-guided aspiration of a lesion yielded pus from which *S. milleri* was grown. Histology showed no evidence of malignancy. After four weeks of antibiotics, a repeat CT scan showed resolution of the liver lesions and she was discharged, apparently cured. One month later she was readmitted with recurrence of symptoms. A large empyema was found in the right hemithorax, which required rib resection to drain. After a stormy course, she finally made a complete recovery.

Why was the patient initially misdiagnosed as having malignant disease?

Which microorganisms may cause liver abscess?

How should liver abscess be managed?

Why did this patient not respond fully to antibiotic therapy?

Background

This case highlights various issues associated with liver abscess, an underconsidered differential diagnosis in patients presenting with non-specific symptoms such as fever, general malaise, fatigue, anorexia and weight loss (Figure 29.1). Pain is frequently absent and 'liver function tests' may be normal.

The white blood cell count and C-reactive protein (CRP) are usually raised, and blood cultures are positive in about half of cases, but the cornerstone of diagnosis is radiology (Figure 29.2). Abdominal ultrasound will demonstrate hepatic lesions, while contrast-enhanced CT scanning is more specific for abscesses and allows better evaluation of their extent. With both it may sometimes be difficult to distinguish abscesses from necrotic metastases or haemorrhage into hepatic cysts. Scanning using magnetic resonance imaging, though not often helpful in this condition, may be useful with small lesions, inaccessible to percutaneous drainage. Positron emission tomography scanning has little to offer as it will not distinguish inflammatory from malignant lesions, both of which may coexist, and the radiologist will aspirate material from lesions whenever possible and send material for microbiological and histological examination (although the former is sometimes negative due to prior empirical antibiotic therapy).

Microbiologically, there are two quite distinct types of liver abscess: amoebic and bacterial (pyogenic). The former is a common and serious disease in the tropics and subtropics caused by the pathogenic protozoan *Entamoeba histolytica*, following ingestion of cysts in water or food contaminated with faeces. Serology is usually positive at the time of presentation. In temperate climates, liver abscess is a bacterial infection, most often encountered in middle age and beyond, when biliary tract disease, especially cholelithiasis, is the commonest association. Rarer conditions include inflammatory bowel disease, diverticulitis, pancreatitis, gastrointestinal surgery, blunt trauma to the abdomen, and even migration to the liver of foreign bodies such as fish or chicken bones and toothpicks. Diabetes mellitus, cirrhosis and malignant disease have been identified as predisposing factors.

Bacterial abscesses may be solitary or multiple and caused by a single species or a mixture, and many different organisms have been reported as causing sporadic infection. Two are of special importance. The first, as in our case study, is *Streptococcus anginosus* (formerly *S. milleri*), belonging to a taxonomic group of three closely related species. Although a normal inhabitant of the gastrointestinal tract between mouth and anus, it possesses an impressive array of virulence factors and toxins, and is capable of causing invasive infections in several body sites. Isolation of *S. anginosus* from blood cultures should always prompt a search for a septic focus, usually intra-abdominal or pelvic, with hepatic abscess high on the list.

Second, in the Far East, strains of *Klebsiella pneumoniae* (especially serotype K1, increasingly multiply antibiotic resistant) have emerged over the last 20 years as important causes of liver abscess, sometimes causing particularly aggressive infections with spread to other

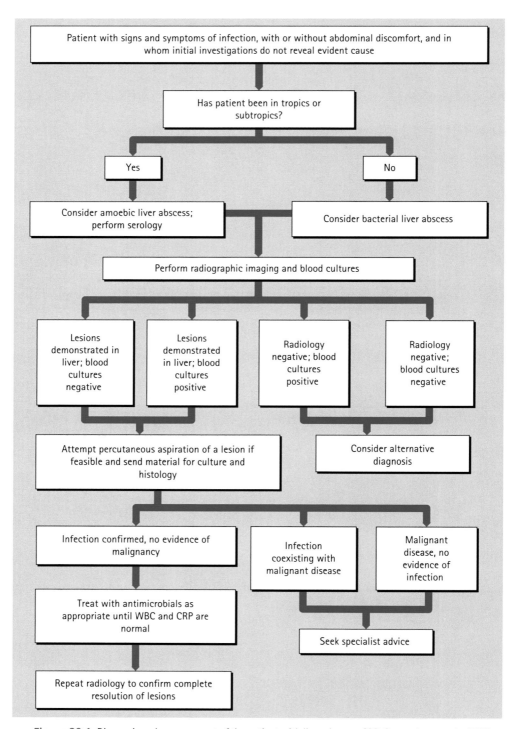

Figure 29.1 Diagnosis and management of the patient with liver abscess. CRP, C-reactive protein; WBC, white blood cell count.

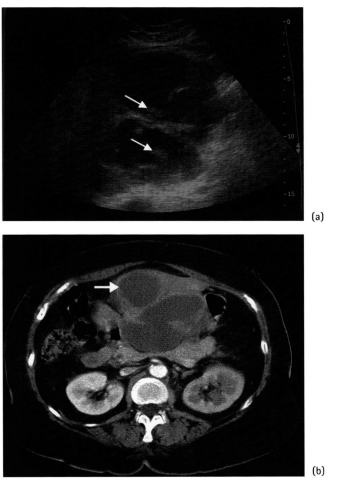

(a)

(b)

Figure 29.2 (a) Transverse ultrasound image in the epigastrium showing fluid collections in the left lobe of the liver (note posterior enhancement). Thick walls and echogenic material within the fluid (arrows), indicating haemorrhage, necrotic material or thick pus, excludes simple cysts. **(b)** Axial CT image, after intravenous contrast, through the upper abdomen in the same patient as in (a) showing the fluid collections expanding the left lobe of the liver. The thin rim of enhancing tissue around the fluid (arrow) is indicative of an abscess.

organs, including the lung, eye and brain. This 'new' disease is currently rare in the UK and Europe, but is occasionally encountered in the USA and Australia.

Mixed infections usually involve two or more gastrointestinal bacteria, typically *Escherichia coli*, enterococci and various anaerobes.

Management

Amoebic abscesses are treated with metronidazole or tinidazole for up to ten days, followed by a ten-day course of diloxanide furoate, which eradicates gut carriage. Aspiration of the abscess, which is usually single, is indicated if response is slow, or imminent rupture is suspected. The prognosis is excellent.

In the case of bacterial abscesses, early drainage is desirable, although cure can sometimes be achieved with antibiotic therapy alone, which may be the only option where there are multiple small abscesses. Drainage is done by CT-guided percutaneous aspiration whenever feasible, and although reports testify to the adequacy of simple needle aspiration (often needing to be repeated), the insertion of a drain is less traumatic for the patient, more convenient for the radiology department, and allows washing out of the abscess cavity, which is especially valuable when pus is thick and difficult to aspirate.

Choice of antibiotics will depend on the knowledge or otherwise of the pathogen(s). *S. anginosus* should be treated with intravenous penicillin (vancomycin for the penicillin-allergic patient), with the addition of gentamicin for the first two weeks or so. The isolation of *E. coli* or an anaerobe from pus or blood suggests the possibility of a mixed aetiology, and in these cases, or when cultures are negative, a combination of antibiotics such as amoxicillin, gentamicin and metronidazole is indicated, to cover all likely possibilities. Amoxicillin might be replaced by a broader-spectrum agent such as piperacillin-tazobactam or a carbapenem for patients with recent hospitalization, in whom the Gram-negative flora of the gut could be multiply resistant to antibiotics. This would also be the case where the causal pathogen was known to be multiply resistant *Klebsiella*, for example. Duration of therapy will depend on response, as indicated by a return to normal of the white blood cell count and CRP, and radiological resolution of the lesion(s), but typically several weeks' therapy is required. Prognosis depends partly on the underlying predisposing factors, which should be thoroughly investigated as part of the management.

Treatment failed in our patient because one of the abscesses had eroded through the diaphragm and produced an empyema in the right hemithorax which was not detected by CT scanning. This is unlikely to be a problem using modern radiological techniques.

Recent Developments

It is likely that liver abscesses caused by virulent and resistant *Klebsiella pneumoniae* strains will become more frequent as these organisms spread worldwide.

Conclusion

Liver abscess continues to pose diagnostic and therapeutic challenges. The message is to retain a 'high index of suspicion' and consider the diagnosis in any patient with non-specific symptoms and signs of occult infection.

Acknowledgement

The author is indebted to Dr Clifford Murch, Consultant Radiologist, for invaluable advice and for the illustrations.

Further Reading

Athavale NV, Leitch DG, Cowling P. Liver abscesses due to Fusobacterium spp that mimic malignant metastatic liver disease. *Eur J Clin Microb Infect Dis* 2002; **21**: 884–6.

Braiteh F, Golden MP. Cryptogenic invasive *Klebsiella pneumoniae* liver abscess syndrome. *Int J Infect Dis* 2007; **11**: 16–22.

Corredoira J, Casariego E, Moreno C *et al.* Prospective study of *Streptococcus milleri* hepatic abscess. *Eur J Clin Micro Infect Dis* 1998; **17**: 556–60.

Indik JH, Masters L. What appears to be cancer. *Arch Intern Med* 1998; **158**: 1374–7.

Lederman ER, Crum NF. Pyogenic liver abscess with a focus on *Klebsiella pneumoniae* as a primary pathogen: an emerging disease with unique clinical characteristics. *Am J Gastroenterol* 2005; **100**: 322–31.

Mohsen AH, Green ST, Read RC, McKendrick MW. Liver abscess in adults: ten years experience in a UK centre. *QJM* 2002; **95**: 797–802.

Mortelé KJ, Segatto E, Ros PR. The infected liver: radiologic-pathologic correlation. *Radiographics* 2004; **24**: 937–55.

Rajak CL, Gupta S, Jain S, Chawla Y, Gulati M, Suri S. Percutaneous treatment of liver abscesses: needle aspiration versus catheter drainage. *Am J Roentgenol* 1998; **170**: 1035–9.

Ryan RS, Al-Hashimi H, Lee MJ. Hepatic abscesses in elderly patients mimicking metastatic disease. *Ir J Med Sci* 2001; **170**: 251–3.

Sridharan GV, Wilkinson SP, Primrose WR. Pyogenic liver abscess in the elderly. *Age Ageing* 1990; **19**: 199–203.

Wang CL, Guo XJ, Qiu SB *et al.* Diagnosis of bacterial hepatic abscess by CT. *Hepatobiliary Pancreat Dis Int* 2007; **6**: 271–5.

PROBLEM

30 *Clostridium difficile*-associated Diarrhoea

Alisdair A. MacConnachie

Case History

 A 72-year-old woman presented to the accident and emergency department with profuse watery diarrhoea and abdominal cramps of three days duration. She had a past medical history of chronic obstructive pulmonary disease and had been discharged from hospital seven days earlier following treatment for an exacerbation of her airways disease. During her previous admission she remembered receiving intravenous antibiotics. As there was concern about the risk of *Clostridium difficile*-associated diarrhoea she was transferred to a single room and commenced on oral metronidazole. Blood testing showed a raised white blood cell count at $25 \times 10^9/l$, a urea of 22 mmol/l and creatinine of 252 µmol/l. Abdominal X-ray did not show toxic dilatation of her colon. The following day her stool toxin assay confirmed the presence of *C. difficile* toxin and she continued on her metronidazole. Over the next three days her diarrhoea settled and she was discharged home on day seven of her admission to complete a further three days of metronidazole.

What risk factors did this lady have for developing *C. difficile*–associated diarrhoea?

On her initial admission, what indicators of severe disease did this lady have, and should they have had implications for her treatment?

What is the risk of her having recurrent disease and, if she does, how could this be treated?

Background

Clostridium difficile is a Gram-positive anaerobic bacillus that was first described as the predominant cause of antibiotic-associated diarrhoea in 1978. Although existing in a vegetative state within the bowel, *C. difficile* produces spores. These spores are stable in the environment for many weeks and resistant to many environmental conditions, cleaning products and antibiotics. Once ingested, they germinate within the colon and, given the correct colonic conditions, can cause disease. The organism produces two toxins that disrupt enterocyte architecture and cause colitis.

The 'normal' colonic microflora control *C. difficile* colonization and prevent disease, therefore anything that disrupts this control reduces resistance to *C. difficile* colonization. The most potent risk for this is the administration of antibiotics to treat other infections (e.g. urinary tract infection, pneumonia). In general, any antibiotic can predispose an individual to *C. difficile*-associated diarrhoea (CDAD) but broad-spectrum agents and those likely to do most damage to the indigenous flora are most closely linked to CDAD. Initially clindamycin was implicated but, more recently, broad-spectrum penicillins, cephalosporins and fluoroquinolones have been implicated. Therefore, both disruption of the colonic microflora and colonization of the colon with *C. difficile* are required in order to get disease. Thus, the main risk factors for CDAD are hospitalization and recent antibiotics.

In recent years there has been a change in the epidemiology of the disease, with several large outbreaks in North America and Europe highlighting more prevalent and severe CDAD with a higher risk of relapse. This has been largely associated with the evolution of a newer strain identified as ribotype 027. This strain of *C. difficile* is resistant to fluoroquinolones (reflecting evolved resistance against antibiotics commonly used in the hospital setting), produces higher levels of toxin and is thus often associated with more severe disease.

Clinical manifestations and diagnosis

C. difficile causes a spectrum of illness ranging from asymptomatic carriage to pseudomembranous colitis and life-threatening fulminant colitis. Around 3% of adults are asymptomatic carriers of *C. difficile* and although as many as 21% of patients will be colonized with *C. difficile* after admission to hospital only 37% of these will be symptomatic with diarrhoea. The reasons why some people are able to carry *C. difficile* asymptomatically are not clear but may reflect the humoral response and the activity of other colonic microflora. CDAD typically presents with loose watery stool, lower abdominal pain, low-grade fever and a slight rise in white blood cell count. This will often occur during or within several days of stopping antibiotics.

 C. difficile can cause more severe disease including pseudomembranous colitis and life-threatening fulminant colitis. Both manifestations result from severe ulceration of the colonic mucosa by *C. difficile*-associated toxin. The clinical findings of abdominal distension, sepsis syndrome, ileus and significant colonic dilatation (>7 cm) should alert the physician to these manifestations. These patients will require more intensive treatment and possibly surgical intervention.

Following clinical suspicion, *C. difficile* is diagnosed by the identification of toxin in stool samples. Although culture can be employed this is technically demanding and takes several days to obtain results. Also, given the high levels of asymptomatic carriage, culture is less indicative of disease than toxin identification. Most laboratories now use an enzyme-linked immunoassay to identify toxin in stool samples. This test has the advantage of obtaining a result within 24 hours but, despite having high specificity, sensitivity can vary from 60% to 95% depending on the test used. Therefore, in patients in whom there is a high clinical suspicion of CDAD, more than one negative toxin assay should be obtained before the diagnosis is dismissed. The older cytotoxin assay remains the gold standard but slow turnaround times and the need for tissue culture make this test less practical.

Imaging modalities may help assess disease severity. Abdominal pain, distension, tenderness or sepsis should prompt abdominal X-ray to exclude colonic dilatation. Computed tomography scanning will often show a pancolitis with colonic wall thickening. Although colonoscopy can demonstrate pseudomembranes, this technique is potentially dangerous as the risk of colonic perforation is high.

Clinical management of CDAD

This involves three crucial steps: general management, assessment of severity, and specific therapy against *C. difficile* (Figure 30.1). Treatment of CDAD should commence as soon as there is sufficient clinical suspicion and not await the results of stool toxin analysis. There is concern that once the colon is awash with toxin, antibiotics may be less useful, and these can always be stopped if toxin analysis is negative. Patients should have the causative antibiotic stopped or, if this is not possible, consideration should be given to narrowing the spectrum. Strict infection control procedures should be followed, with the patient managed in a single room and all staff observing hand hygiene precautions with the use of gloves and aprons and hand-washing with soap and water. *C. difficile* spores are alcohol resistant and therefore the use of alcohol hand rubs is not appropriate. There are natural concerns about the use of antimotility agents in patients with CDAD and, although the evidence of harm is inconclusive, consideration should be given to stopping these.

Oral metronidazole or vancomycin should be commenced and stool collected for toxin analysis. Early antibiotic administration is unlikely to affect stool toxin results as these tests do not assess the presence of viable organisms. Intravenous metronidazole does achieve clinically useful colonic levels and is useful when the oral route is compromised

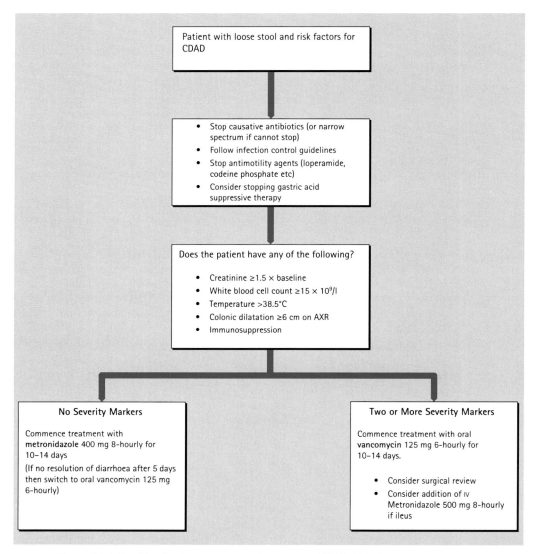

Patient with loose stool and risk factors for CDAD

- Stop causative antibiotics (or narrow spectrum if cannot stop)
- Follow infection control guidelines
- Stop antimotility agents (loperamide, codeine phosphate etc)
- Consider stopping gastric acid suppressive therapy

Does the patient have any of the following?

- Creatinine ≥1.5 × baseline
- White blood cell count ≥15 × 10⁹/l
- Temperature >38.5°C
- Colonic dilatation ≥6 cm on AXR
- Immunosuppression

No Severity Markers

Commence treatment with **metronidazole** 400 mg 8-hourly for 10–14 days
(If no resolution of diarrhoea after 5 days then switch to oral vancomycin 125 mg 6-hourly)

Two or More Severity Markers

Commence treatment with oral **vancomycin** 125 mg 6-hourly for 10–14 days.

- Consider surgical review
- Consider addition of IV Metronidazole 500 mg 8-hourly if ileus

Figure 30.1 Algorithm for the assessment and treatment of CDAD. AXR, abdominal X-ray; IV, intravenous.

or there are concerns about oral drug delivery such as in paralytic ileus. Intravenous vancomycin does not achieve adequate colonic levels and should not be used to treat CDAD. In non-severe disease, metronidazole and vancomycin have equal efficacy and, due to a variety of factors, metronidazole is preferred. In severe disease, oral vancomycin may be superior, possibly relating to the predictable colonic levels achieved as it is not absorbed from the gastrointestinal tract. Therefore, prior to commencing antibiotics, there needs to be an assessment of the severity of the patient's illness. There is no universally accepted definition of severe CDAD; however, several factors have been shown to correlate with a more complicated illness. These include raised white blood cell count, renal dysfunction, fever, hypoalbuminaemia, colonic dilatation and sepsis syndrome. Treatment is usually for 10 to 14 days but duration will be guided by clinical response and more prolonged courses are occasionally necessary. In severe disease, clinicians should have a low threshold for seeking surgical involvement as patients with fulminant colitis or those unresponsive to medical therapy may benefit from subtotal colectomy.

Control of CDAD

Control of *C. difficile* requires both implementation of strict hand hygiene and isolation procedures as well as vigilance in antibiotic prescribing policy and practice. Restricting volume of prescribing (number and duration of antibiotic courses) and the types of agents used (in particular the broad-spectrum penicillin–β-lactamase inhibitor combinations, cephalosporins and fluoroquinolones) has been associated with significant reductions in CDAD. A continued commitment to antimicrobial stewardship combined with strict implementation of infection control procedures should see a continued reduction in the incidence of CDAD.

Recent Developments

Following a first episode of CDAD, up to 40% of patients will relapse. Relapse (following complete cessation of loose stools) is not associated with resistance to metronidazole or vancomycin but likely represents either environmental re-infection or persistence (and germination) of colonic spores. It is therefore recommended that first relapses are re-treated with the same regimen. Following one relapse, the risk of subsequent relapse

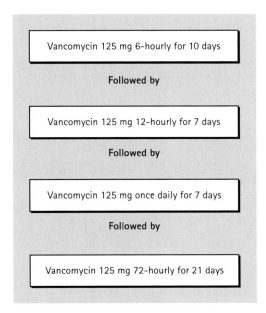

Figure 30.2 Pulsed and tapered vancomycin.

increases to up to 65% and treatment should be with vancomycin dosed in a pulsed and tapered manner (Figure 30.2). Intermittent dosing of vancomycin allows spores the chance to germinate and thus become antibiotic susceptible. Management of further relapses is less well delineated. Therapies used include the administration of pooled human immunoglobulin, toxin-binding resins, newer antimicrobial agents and faecal bacteriotherapy. Faecal bacteriotherapy – the administration of donor faeces via enema, at colonoscopy, or nasogastric tube – has had the most successful results in small, observational cohorts of patients with recurrent disease. These treatments do, however, suffer from aesthetic problems and the screening of donors and preparation of the donor stool are cumbersome and time consuming. As these treatments become refined they may produce a truly viable option for individuals who have failed to settle on all other treatments. An impaired humoral immune response to infection is a feature of severe and recurrent disease. Early studies with vaccination suggest that this may be a useful modality for prevention and treatment of CDAD.

Conclusion

CDAD is a serious debilitating and potentially life-threatening healthcare associated infection. Early recognition and empirical therapy, pending confirmatory investigations, is essential to optimise outcome. Treatment should be stratified to the severity of the infection.

Further Reading

Aas J, Gessert CE, Bakken JS. Recurrent *Clostridium difficile* colitis: case series involving 18 patients treated with donor stool administered via a nasogastric tube. *Clin Infect Dis* 2003; **36**: 580–5.

Bartlett, JG, Moon N, Chang TW, Taylor N, Onderdonk AB. Role of *Clostridium difficile* in antibiotic-associated pseudomembranous colitis. *Gastroenterology* 1978; **75**: 778–82.

Bartlett JG. Narrative review: the new epidemic of *Clostridium difficile*-associated enteric disease. *Ann Intern Med* 2006; **145**: 758–64.

McFarland LV, Mulligan ME, Kwok RY, Stamm WE. Nosocomial acquisition of *Clostridium difficile* infection. *N Engl J Med* 1989; **320**: 204–10.

McFarland LV, Elmer GW, Surawicz CM. Breaking the cycle: treatment strategies for 163 cases of recurrent *Clostridium difficile* disease. *Am J Gastroenterol* 2002; **97**: 1769–75.

Pépin J, Valiquette L, Alary ME *et al. Clostridium difficile*-associated diarrhea in a region of Quebec from 1991 to 2003: a changing pattern of disease severity. *CMAJ* 2004; **171**: 466–72.

31 Bloody Diarrhoea (*E. coli* O157)

Stephanie Dundas

Case History

A 67-year-old woman was admitted to the surgical ward with a 72-hour history of increasingly severe abdominal pain and bloody diarrhoea. The referral from the general practitioner indicated a known history of diverticular disease, hypertension and ischaemic heart disease. Her medications included aspirin, an angiotensin-converting enzyme inhibitor, a β blocker and a proton pump inhibitor. Examination confirmed marked left-sided abdominal tenderness, guarding and a slight tachycardia but otherwise was normal. Initial routine blood tests revealed a neutrophilia but were otherwise unremarkable. She was managed presumptively for diverticular disease with intravenous fluids and antibiotics. On the day after her admission her renal function tests indicated a significant rise in urea and creatinine.

What is the most likely diagnosis and what complication may she be developing?

Which investigations would you request next?

How should she be managed?

What is her prognosis?

Background

In the elderly patient presenting with severe abdominal pain and bloody diarrhoea, surgical pathologies are often considered first and infections may be overlooked. Although inflammatory bowel disease, diverticulitis and mesenteric ischaemia are within the differential diagnosis, the commonest cause of bloody diarrhoea, irrespective of age, is infectious gastroenteritis. The most common infection is Campylobacter; Salmonella infections are significantly less common and *Escherichia coli* O157:H7 infections are comparatively rare. *E. coli* O157 infection usually presents as a self-limiting haemorrhagic colitis; however, about 15% of infections will be complicated by the development of the haemolytic uraemic syndrome (HUS).

HUS is defined by the following characteristic triad:

1   Anaemia (haematocrit <30%) with red blood cell (RBC) destruction on blood film
2   Thrombocytopenia (platelet count <150 × 10^9/l)
3   Acute renal failure (creatinine level greater than the upper limit of normal for age)

HUS is much more common at the extremes of age, and young children and the elderly have a fourfold higher risk of developing HUS. HUS is an evolving process and on average it is 7 days (range 5–13 days) from the onset of diarrhoea before the syndrome is fully established (Figure 31.1). There are, however, clear differences – usually from the beginning – between patients who go on to get HUS and those in whom *E. coli* O157 infection resolves without complication. Patients who develop HUS usually have a very high white blood cell count (WCC) on admission and, equally, those with a normal WCC are unlikely to get HUS. Fragmented RBCs on the blood film accompanied by a rise in lactate dehydrogenase (LDH) are also early features of HUS and usually these changes precede the rise in creatinine, thrombocytopenia and anaemia which define the syndrome. Although acute renal failure is the commonest clinical manifestation of HUS, neurological complications – particularly confusion, seizures and cerebrovascular accidents – are also common.

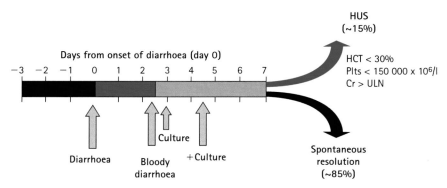

Figure 31.1 Clinical course of *E. coli* O157:H7 infection (adapted with permission from Tarr PI, Gordon C, Chandler W. Shiga-toxin-producing *Escherichia coli* and haemolytic uraemic syndrome. *Lancet* 2005; **365**:1073–86). Cr, creatinine; HCT, haematocrit; Plts, platelets; ULN, upper limit of normal.

In *E. coli* O157 infection, HUS is caused by a specific exotoxin. The nomenclature is confusing with the toxin known as verocytotoxin or more usually Shiga toxin, because it is identical to the toxin released by *Shigella dysenteriae* serotype 1. Other exotoxin-producing *E. coli* (e.g. serotypes O26, O145 and O104) have been called both verocytotoxin-producing (VTEC) and Shiga toxin-producing (STEC) *E. coli*. The process by which STEC cause HUS is not completely understood. The organism attaches to the gut epithelial cells and releases Shiga toxin, which is presumably absorbed into the circulation, although it has never been detected in blood. Pro-inflammatory cytokines are released and Shiga toxin binds to specific GB3 cell receptors, which leads to endocytosis of the toxin. The primary injury is vascular endothelial damage which is followed by thrombotic occlusion of capillaries and swelling, apoptosis and necrosis of cells. GB3 receptors are predominant in kidneys and the brain and this is thought to explain the renal and neurological complications of HUS. Interactions between Shiga toxin and circulating leukocytes and platelets may also have a role in the pathogenesis.

Case discussion

In a patient presenting with bloody diarrhoea and deteriorating renal function, *E. coli* O157 complicated by HUS should be considered as a probable diagnosis. A detailed food history, enquiry about contacts and involvement of Public Health are essential in these circumstances. The patient described was confirmed to have *E. coli* O157 infection on stool culture, the result of which was available two days after her admission. She was transferred to the Infectious Diseases Unit and managed in a single room.

Investigations required to make the diagnosis of HUS are a full blood count, blood film, urea and electrolytes, LDH (which is a quantitative marker of RBC haemolysis) and a coagulation screen. On the day after her admission, this patient's creatinine was 170 μmol/l, platelet count 110×10^9/l, LDH 1600 U/l and haemoglobin 11 g/dl. A coagulation screen was normal, as is usually the case in HUS, and this can be used to distinguish HUS from disseminated intravascular coagulation, which is associated with prolonged coagulation but otherwise has similar laboratory features to HUS. All bloods should be monitored daily until the platelet count begins to rise when the period of highest risk of progressive renal failure is over.

This patient continued to pass urine at 40 ml/hr and treatment with plasma exchange was initiated. Plasma exchange is controversial in the context of *E. coli* O157-associated HUS but it may have a role in the early stages, particularly in adults who have a higher incidence of neurological complications associated with HUS and consequently have a clinical picture more closely related to thrombotic thrombocytopenic purpura. Dialysis remains the cornerstone of treatment in HUS associated with oliguria/anuria and deteriorating renal function and about 50% of patients with HUS will require dialysis.

Recent Developments

HUS can only really be prevented by preventing STEC infections. In terms of reducing the risk of HUS after infection, there is evidence that patients who are admitted earlier and receive intravenous fluids earlier have reduced risk of HUS and it may be that volume expansion is important in reducing risk. After volume restoration, fluid replacement must proceed cautiously as patients may be developing renal failure, they have additional problems of leaky capillaries and low albumin (which can result in fluid in the wrong places), and pulmonary oedema is not uncommon. There is no evidence that antibiotics are beneficial in STEC infections and some evidence to suggest that they are associated with increased risk of HUS and should therefore be avoided. Similarly, antimotility drugs and non-steroidal anti-inflammatory drugs have been associated with HUS and they should not be used.

In the elderly patient with HUS, mortality rates are high, perhaps as high as 50% even with dialysis and intensive management. Neurological and cardiovascular complications of HUS are responsible for much of the mortality in this age group. Mortality rates in children have improved dramatically in recent years, largely due to improved dialysis techniques, and are now less than 10%.

Non O157 serotypes are of increasing concern. Between May and June 2011, the largest ever recorded outbreak of STEC causing HUS was recorded in Germany. The outbreak was caused by the O104 serotype and over 2000 people were affected. High rates of HUS were observed in adults outwith the typical 'at risk' age range.

Conclusion

HUS is a serious and life-threatening complication of *E. coli* O157 infection. Our understanding of the pathology, management and outcomes of HUS is evolving; however, there are still unanswered questions, particularly why children and the elderly are predisposed, why Shiga toxin has never been detected in blood and on the role of plasma exchange in the treatment of adult patients. The emergence of non-O104 serotypes with the potential to cause large outbreaks is of concern and currently not clearly understood.

Further Reading

Chandler WL, Jelacic S, Boster DR *et al.* Prothrombotic coagulation abnormalities preceding the haemolytic-uremic syndrome. *N Engl J Med* 2002; **346**: 23–32.

Dundas S, Murphy J, Soutar RL, Jones GA, Hutchinson SJ, Todd WT. Effectiveness of therapeutic plasma exchange in the 1996 Lanarkshire *Escherichia coli* O157:H7 outbreak. *Lancet* 1999; **354**: 1327–30.

Dundas S, Todd WT, Stewart AI, Murdoch PS, Chaudhuri AK, Hutchison SJ. The central Scotland *Escherichia coli* O157:H7 outbreak: risk factors for the hemolytic uremic syndrome and death among hospitalized patients. *Clin Infect Dis* 2001; **33**: 923–31.

Frank C, Faber M, Askar M, Bernard H, Fruth A, Gilsdorf A. Large and ongoing outbreak of haemolytic uraemic syndrome, Germany, May 2011. *Euro Surveill* 2011; **16**: pii: 19878.

Karmali MA, Steele BT, Petric M, Lim C. Sporadic cases of haemolytic-uraemic syndrome associated with faecal cytotoxin and cytotoxin-producing *Escherichia coli* in stools. *Lancet* 1983; **1**: 619–20.

Te Loo DM, Monnens LA, van Der Velden TJ *et al.* Binding and transfer of verocytotoxin by polymorphonuclear leukocytes in hemolytic uremic syndrome. *Blood* 2000; **95**: 3396–402.

Wong CS, Jelacic S, Habeeb RL, Watkins SL, Tarr PI. The risk of the hemolytic-uremic syndrome after antibiotic treatment of *Escherichia coli* O157:H7 infections. *N Engl J Med* 2000; **342**: 1930–6.

COMMUNITY–ACQUIRED BLOODSTREAM INFECTIONS

PROBLEM

32 Meningococcal Meningitis

Christopher Duncan

Case History

A 36-year-old woman was admitted with sudden-onset severe occipital headache, photophobia and vomiting. On physical examination she was afebrile, with obvious photophobia and neck stiffness but no skin rashes. She was commenced on intravenous

(IV) ceftriaxone, and due to concern about possible subarachnoid haemorrhage she underwent an emergency computed tomography scan of the brain (normal) prior to lumbar puncture (LP). LP demonstrated a neutrophil leukocytosis, raised protein and low glucose, and Gram stain revealed Gram-negative diplococci. Cerebrospinal fluid (CSF) culture was negative. At day five she became breathless with a resting tachycardia, elevated jugular venous pressure, pulsus paradoxus and pericardial rub. Clinical diagnosis of pericardial tamponade was confirmed on echocardiogram and urgent pericardiocentesis was performed.

Why did the organisms seen in CSF fail to culture, and what other options are there for diagnosis?

What was the possible cause for the pericardial effusion, and should treatment be altered?

What are the public health implications?

Background

Neisseria meningitidis is the second commonest cause of community-acquired bacterial meningitis amongst adults, and the commonest cause amongst children in the developed world. Epidemic or sporadic infections occur, in some cases progressing rapidly from onset of symptoms to death in a matter of hours. The greatest burden of meningococcal disease remains in the developing world, particularly the 'Meningitis Belt' of Sub-Saharan Africa where large epidemics frequently occur.

The British Infection Society has produced guidelines for the early management of meningococcal disease in adults (Figure 32.1) These recommend IV ceftriaxone 2 g bid after blood cultures have been obtained. Administration of antibiotic should only be delayed prior to LP if this can be performed within 30 minutes of hospital admission. Supportive treatment includes IV fluids, oxygen supplementation and vasopressors if required. Adjunctive corticosteroid, although helpful in pneumococcal meningitis, is of no significant benefit in meningococcal meningitis, and should be discontinued when the diagnosis of meningococcal infection is made. Antibiotic therapy should be modified to IV benzylpenicillin when CSF culture results demonstrate susceptibility to penicillin. It should be noted that the incidence of penicillin resistance amongst meningococcal isolates remains low in the UK.

The prognosis of meningococcal disease has not improved significantly since the 1960s, despite vast improvements in supportive management and critical care. Current mortality rates remain between 10% and 14% in the USA and approximately 6% in the UK. The most significant predictor of mortality is delay in antibiotic therapy. In a large prospective study in Barcelona, pre-hospital antibiotic administration was associated with a significant reduction in mortality in meningococcal disease (Barquet *et al.*, 1997). Pre-hospital intramuscular benzylpenicillin is therefore recommended in suspected meningococcal disease. In this study other independent predictors of mortality were disseminated intravascular coagulation (DIC), focal neurological deficits and age >60 years.

Early Recognition

- Petechial/purpuric non-blanching rash or signs of meningitis
- A rash may be absent or atypical at presentation
- Neck stiffness may be absent in up to 30% of cases of meningitis
- Prior antibiotics may mask the severity of the illness

Assess Severity & Immediate Intervention[a]

- Airway
- Breathing - respiratory rate & O$_2$ saturation
- Circulation - pulse; capillary refill time (hypotension late); urine output
- Mental status (deterioration may be a sign of shock or meningitis)
- Neurology – focal neurological signs; persistent seizures; papilloedema

Secure Airway
High Flow O$_2$
Large bore IV cannula ± fluid resuscitation

Priority Investigations:
FBC; U+Es; blood sugar, LFTs; CRP
Clotting profile
Blood gases

Microbiology:
Blood culture
Throat swab
Clotted blood
EDTA blood for PCR

Predominantly Meningococcal Septicaemia

- Do not attempt LP
- IV 2g cefotaxime or ceftriaxone
- Call critical care team for review

Predominantly Meningitis[b,c,d]

- Assess patient carefully before performing LP
- Call critical care team if any features of raised ICP, shock or respiratory failure
- If uncertain ask for senior review
- Monitor and stabilize circulation

Signs of Shock[a]
YES   NO

**No Signs of Shock
No Raised ICP
No Respiratory Failure[a,b]**

Signs of Raised ICP[a,b]

Priorities

Secure airway + High flow O$_2$
Volume resuscitation
Senior review
Management in critical care unit

Lumbar Puncture[a,b]

- IV 2g cefotaxime/ ceftriaxone immediately after LP
- Consider corticosteroids[d]
- If LP will be delayed for more than 30 minutes give IV antibiotics first

Priorities

- Secure airway + High flow O$_2$
- Defer lumbar puncture
- IV 2g cefotaxime/ceftriaxone
- Consider corticosteroids[d]
- Careful volume resuscitation
- 30° head elevation
- Management in critical care unit
- Low threshold for elective Intubation + ventilation (cerebral protection)

No Improvement

Improvement

Further Interventions

Pre-emptive intubation + ventilation
Volume support
Inotropic/vasopressor support
Manage in critical care environment

Careful Monitoring[a] Repeated Review

Additional Information

[a]Warning signs
The following warn of impending/ worsening shock, respiratory failure or raised ICP and require urgent senior review and intervention (see algorithm):

- Rapidly progressive rash
- Poor peripheral perfusion, CRT >4 secs, oliguria and systolic BP <90 (hypotension often a late sign)
- RR <8 or >30
- Pulse rate <40 or >140
- Acidosis pH <7.3 or BE worse than –5
- WBC <4
- Marked depressed conscious level (GCS <12) or a fluctuating conscious level (falling GCS >2)
- Focal neurology
- Persistent seizures
- Bradycardia and hypertension
- Papilloedema

[b]CT scan and meningitis
This investigation should only be used when appropriate:

- A normal CT scan does not exclude raised ICP
- If there are no clinical contraindictions to LP, a CT scan is not necessary beforehand
- Subsequently a CT scan may be useful in identifying dural defects predisposing to meningitis

[c]Appropriate antibiotics for bacterial meningitis
Review with microbiology:

- Ampicillin IV 2g qds should be added for individuals >55 years to cover Listeria
- Vancomycin ± rifampicin if pneumococcal penicillin resistance suspected
- Amend antibiotics on the basis of microbiology results

[d]Corticosteroids in adult meningitis

- Dexamethasone 0.15 mg/kg qds for 4 days started with or just before the first dose of antibiotics, particularly where pneumococcal meningitis suspected
- Do not give unless you are confident you are using the correct antimicrobials
- Stop the dexamethasone if a non-

When antibiotics have been administered prior to LP, the CSF is rapidly sterilized, often within 3–4 hours. In the event of negative cultures there are other options available for diagnosis:

- Polymerase chain reaction (PCR) is a sensitive and rapid tool for diagnosing meningococcal infection, and is less affected by prior antibiotic exposure than culture. PCR can be performed on CSF and serum, and should be requested in all cases if available. PCR does not give information about antimicrobial susceptibility.
- Latex agglutination kits, which identify meningococcal capsular antigens, are available for use in CSF and urine. These kits detect agglutination of five capsular types: A, B, C, Y and W135. Unfortunately, the sensitivity for serotype B (the commonest cause of infections in the UK) is low.

PCR of CSF in this case was positive for *N. meningitidis* serotype B.

Several complications are associated with meningococcal disease. The main concerns are septic shock and DIC, which require management in a critical care environment. Other major complications necessitating specific therapy include:

- Acute respiratory distress syndrome
- Neurological complications including coma (usually secondary to cerebral oedema or obstructive hydrocephalus), seizures and/or focal neurological deficits
- Arthritis (septic or reactive)
- Pericarditis

Pericarditis in meningococcal disease arises from two mechanisms. Primary pericardial infection, resulting in purulent pericarditis, is a rare manifestation of meningococcal disease. More commonly, as in the case above, immunologically mediated reactive pericarditis can occur, leading to pericardial effusion (Figure 32.2). In both situations pericardial tamponade can develop, necessitating urgent drainage.

Although infection amongst contacts of a case of meningococcal disease is rare, the attack rate amongst close contacts of patients with infection is significantly higher (500–800 times) than the general population. Chemoprophylaxis should therefore be administered to close contacts (defined as household or 'kissing contacts') as soon as possible after identification of the index case, and ideally within 24 hours. The case should be notified to the Consultant in Public Health Medicine, who can advise on choice and duration of chemoprophylaxis. Healthcare workers do not require chemoprophylaxis unless there has been direct contact with oral secretions (during mouth-to-mouth ventilation or endotracheal intubation). Various options are available, and traditionally, rifampicin was the agent of choice. Single-dose ciprofloxacin is now usually recommended for both non-pregnant adults and children, with ceftriaxone recommended during pregnancy.

Figure 32.1 British Infection Society Guidelines on the management of meningococcal disease in immunocompetent adults (reproduced with permission). BE, base excess; BP, blood pressure (mmHg); CRP, C-reactive protein; CRT, capillary refill time; CT, computed tomography; EDTA, ethylene diamine tetraacetic acid; FBC, full blood count; GCS, Glasgow Coma Scale; ICP, intracranial pressure; LFTs, liver function tests; PCR, polymerase chain reaction; RR, respiratory rate; U+Es, urea and electrolytes; WBC, white blood cell count (x 10^9/l).

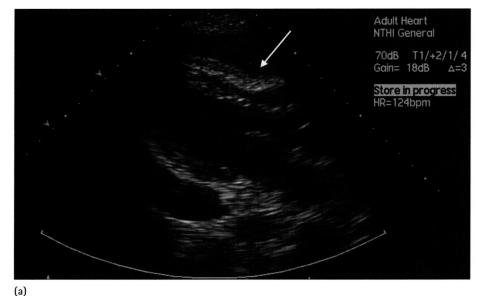

(a)

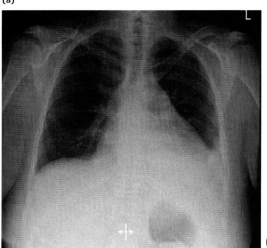

(b)

Figure 32.2 (a) Transthoracic long-axis echocardiogram demonstrating pericardial effusion with diastolic collapse of right ventricle (arrowed), indicating pericardial tamponade. (b) Chest radiograph demonstrating increased cardiac silhouette with obscured left hemidiaphragm consistent with pericardial and left pleural effusions.

Recent Developments

There is evidence that activation of protein C, which has anticoagulant and anti-inflammatory properties, is impaired in severe meningococcal disease. In addition, patients with purpura fulminans, a severe form of DIC resulting in skin necrosis and tissue loss, have lower circulating levels of protein C. A small, randomized, placebo-controlled trial (RCT) of administration of protein C concentrate in severe meningococcal disease in children showed no benefit in terms of reducing mortality or amputation, although administration did improve coagulopathy (de Kleijn *et al.*, 2003). Other small trials have suggested mortality and morbidity benefits (White *et al.*, 2000). Large RCTs are required to assess the role of protein C concentrate in severe meningococcal disease. There are limited data regarding the use of recombinant activated protein C (drotrecogin alpha) in meningococcal disease (Vincent *et al.*, 2005).

Novel therapies, such as a recombinant protein composed of the N-terminal fragment of human bactericidal/permeability-increasing protein (rBPI), which both lyses *N. Meningitidis* and binds to bacterial endotoxin, are under investigation. In a RCT of rBPI versus placebo albumin, involving 393 children with meningococcal disease and petechial or purpuric rashes (Figure 32.3), rBPI was associated with a statistically significant improvement in functional outcome and a trend towards fewer amputations, although no difference in mortality was seen at 60 days.

Vaccination against serotype C *N. meningitidis* is routine in the UK, and has led to a reduction in the incidence of serotype C infections, together with evidence of the development of herd immunity. Research into the development of a serotype B vaccine is ongoing, with two candidate vaccines currently under investigation.

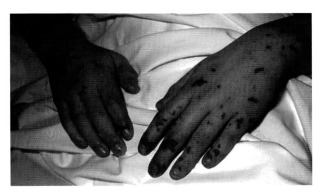

Figure 32.3 Purpuric rash in meningococcal infection (*see inside front cover for colour version*).

Conclusion

Meningococcal meningitis remains a common cause of community-acquired bacterial meningitis with a mortality rate which has remained significant despite improvements in supportive care over 40 years. Rapid administration of appropriate antibiotic therapy remains the most important determinant of good outcome. The development of effective vaccines against all serotypes of *N. meningitidis* remains a priority to reduce the burden of disease in the future.

Further Reading

Barquet N, Domingo P, Caylà JA *et al.* Prognostic factors in meningococcal disease. Development of a bedside predictive model and scoring system. Barcelona Meningococcal Disease Surveillance Group. *JAMA* 1997; **278**: 491–6.

Bilukha OO, Rosenstein N. Prevention and control of meningococcal disease. Recommendations of the Advisory Committee on Immunization Practices (ACIP). *MMWR Recomm Rep* 2005; **54**(RR-7): 1–21.

de Kleijn ED, de Groot R, Hack CE *et al.* Activation of protein C following infusion of protein C concentrate in children with severe meningococcal sepsis and purpura fulminans: a randomized, double-blinded, placebo-controlled, dose-finding study. *Crit Care Med* 2003; **31**: 1839–47.

Gray SJ, Trotter CL, Ramsay ME *et al.* Epidemiology of meningococcal disease in England and Wales 1993/94 to 2003/04: contribution and experiences of the Meningococcal Reference Unit. *J Med Microbiol* 2006; **55**: 887–96.

Heyderman RS, Lambert HP, O'Sullivan I, Stuart JM, Taylor BL, Wall RA. Early management of suspected bacterial meningitis and meningococcal septicaemia in adults. *J Infect* 2003; **46**: 75–7.

Levin M, Quint PA, Goldstein B *et al.* Recombinant bactericidal/permeability-increasing protein (rBPI21) as adjunctive treatment for children with severe meningococcal sepsis: a randomised trial. rBPI21 Meningococcal Sepsis Study Group. *Lancet* 2000; **356**: 961–7.

Stephens DS, Greenwood B, Brandtzaeg P. Epidemic meningitis, meningococcaemia, and Neisseria meningitidis. *Lancet* 2007; **369**: 2196–210.

Vincent JL, Nadel S, Kutsogiannis DJ *et al.* Drotrecogin alfa (activated) in patients with severe sepsis presenting with purpura fulminans, meningitis, or meningococcal disease: a retrospective analysis of patients enrolled in recent clinical studies. *Crit Care* 2005; **9**: R331–43.

White B, Livingstone W, Murphy C, Hodgson A, Rafferty M, Smith OP. An open-label study of the role of adjuvant hemostatic support with protein C replacement therapy in purpura fulminans-associated meningococcemia. *Blood* 2000; **96**: 3719–24.

PROBLEM

33 Necrobacillosis

Beth White

Case History

A previously well 20-year-old male student was admitted with rigors, malaise, neck pain, breathlessness and a dry cough. He had had a sore throat in the last week but had received no antibiotic therapy. On admission he was febrile, tachycardic and tachypnoeic and his oxygen saturations were 92% on room air. He was tender along the distribution of the left sternocleidomastoid muscle with some difficulty flexing and rotating his neck. He had some cervical adenopathy but his throat was not inflamed. Examination was otherwise unremarkable.

Investigations revealed a neutrophil leukocytosis of $18 \times 10^9/l$ and C-reactive protein (CRP) was elevated at 165 mg/l. Transaminases and bilirubin were slightly elevated at 48 U/l and 40 µmol/l, respectively. A chest radiograph was clear but, due to dyspnoea and pleuritic chest pain, computed tomography (CT) of the chest was performed which revealed multiple septic pulmonary emboli. Intravenous drug misuse was denied. Blood cultures subsequently grew *Fusobacterium necrophorum*.

What other investigations might you consider?

What antibiotics would you use to treat this patient?

If you did not have any microbiology data, would this change your antibiotic choice?

How long would you wish to continue antibiotics for?

What complications would you look out for in this patient?

Background

First described in 1936 by Andre Lemierre, a French Professor of Microbiology and Infectious Diseases, Lemierre's syndrome is the classical presentation of human necrobacillosis. The key finding is septicaemia due to *Fusobacterium necrophorum*, an obligate Gram-negative bacterium.

Professor Lemierre described a collection of cases characterized by an initial pharyngotonsillitis or peritonsillar abscess in young, previously healthy persons, followed by septic thrombophlebitis of the internal jugular vein (IJV) and subsequent metastatic embolic abscesses in lung and bones. These were mainly caused by *F. necrophorum*. Mortality was substantial, with 18 of 20 patients dying.

The incidence of Lemierre's syndrome has fallen markedly since the beginning of the antibiotic era, but there has been a small rise in cases over the last few decades. This has provoked comment that cases are linked with a more restricted use of penicillin in primary care for acute tonsillitis. Lemierre's syndrome remains rare, however, with a recent Danish prospective study reporting an incidence of 14.4 cases per million people per year in those aged 15–24 years old (Kristensen and Prag, 2008).

Pathogenesis

The syndrome may be preceded by a viral or bacterial pharyngitis. Approximately 10% of published cases are associated with infectious mononucleosis, which is thought to facilitate invasion of fusiform bacteria. The syndrome can also follow primary dental infection. The infection then extends from the oropharynx to the parapharyngeal space, within which is the carotid sheath (enclosing the IJV, internal carotid artery, vagus nerve and lymph nodes). Endovascular infection of the IJV leads to bacteraemia and metastatic spread. This spread is most commonly to the lungs (in up to 85% of cases), but infection can also embolize to the joints or more rarely to bones or muscles. It can cause intra-abdominal abscesses, meningitis, endocarditis or mediastinitis due to extension along the carotid sheath.

Clinical features

Necrobacillosis is commonly seen in young, normally fit and healthy individuals. Classically, 4–12 days following a sore throat, the patient develops fever and rigors, neck pain (from thrombophlebitis of the IJV) and symptoms and signs of metastatic spread; for example, breathlessness, pleuritic pain or haemoptysis; joint pain or swelling, etc.

In some patients there is retrograde extension of the IJV clot, leading to thrombosis of the sigmoid or cavernous sinus. This produces a headache, occasionally cranial nerve palsies and subsequently increasing confusion and coma. This is a rare but serious complication, and is one of the situations where anticoagulation is used, as discussed below.

Diagnosis

The key to diagnosis is awareness of this rare but life-threatening condition.

Laboratory studies

- There is often neutrophilia and raised CRP. Up to 50% of cases have an elevated bilirubin, and up to 23% of cases can develop low-grade disseminated intravascular coagulation.
- Blood cultures are of key importance and should be performed PRIOR to any antibiotics, since the identification of *F. necrophorum* in blood cultures should prompt immediate consideration of Lemierre's syndrome (Figure 33.1). It should be noted that other pathogens have also been implicated in up to 10% of cases (including other *Fusobacterium* spp., *Bacteroides* spp. and *Streptococcus* spp.) and mixed infections can also occur in up to a third of cases.

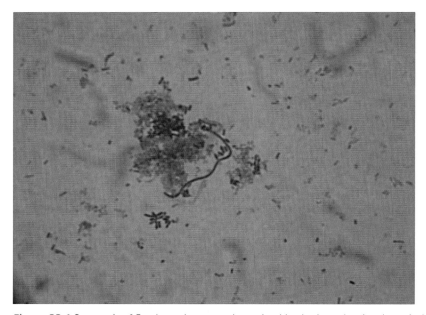

Figure 33.1 Gram stain of *Fusobacterium necrophorum* in a blood culture showing the typical pleiomorphism (courtesy of Dr Jon Brazier from the Anaerobe Reference Laboratory, Cardiff) (*see inside front cover for colour version*).

Imaging

- *Chest radiograph* is often normal, but may show ill-defined infiltrates, or evidence of effusion.
- *CT chest* is strongly recommended, since it is more sensitive for detecting septic emboli, and will pick up abnormalities at an earlier stage than with a simple chest radiograph.
- *Carotid Doppler ultrasound of the neck* is sometimes used to look for evidence of venous thrombosis. It is simple and safe, but is not particularly sensitive, particularly for early thrombus which has little inherent echogenicity.
- *CT neck* is sometimes used instead of carotid Doppler ultrasound, and can also give views of the parapharyngeal space in order to define the extent of any collections or abscesses.

Physicians need to remain alert to the possibility of non-pulmonary metastatic complications and tailor their investigations depending on the symptoms present. They should also have a low threshold for arranging echocardiography.

Treatment

Antibiotics

It is important to obtain blood cultures and other microbiological specimens (for example, from metastatic deposits) in order to guide antibiotic choice most effectively. **Metronidazole** has excellent activity against all strains of *Fusobacterium* spp. It is bactericidal, has a low minimum inhibitory concentration and penetrates well into most tissues. It should not be used alone, however, due to the high incidence of mixed infections. Most experts would therefore recommend combination treatment with **high-dose penicillin** plus **metronidazole**. **Clindamycin** monotherapy can also be very effective, since this antibiotic can be used for patients allergic to penicillin and provides additional anaerobic cover.

The optimal duration of treatment of necrobacillosis has not been firmly established. Due to the endovascular nature of the infection and metastatic complications, prolonged antibiotic therapy is usually required – at least 2–3 weeks of intravenous antibiotics. Providing clinical improvement is seen, it may then be reasonable to switch to oral antibiotics to complete a total of at least six weeks' therapy.

Surgical intervention

It is important to drain abscesses where possible as antibiotics may not be able to penetrate empyema collection and septic arthritis. If recurrent septic embolization occurs despite effective antibiotic therapy, ligation of the IJV can be considered.

Recent Developments

Anticoagulation

Anticoagulation is controversial and papers advocating its use are supported by case reports of small numbers of patients only. It is notable that a lot of this work is in children. It is a procedure that is used more frequently in septic thrombophlebitis of the pelvic veins, but even this practice is not evidence-based, with little benefit over antibiotics alone. At present it is generally reserved for patients in whom there is retrograde extension of the thrombus to the cavernous sinus. This is due to concerns that anticoagulation risks extending the infection, as well as increasing the bleeding risk in patients who often already have multiorgan dysfunction.

Anticoagulation has most commonly been with heparin followed by up to three months of warfarin, but low-molecular-weight heparin has also been used.

Conclusion

 Necrobacillosis is a rare but life-threatening condition affecting previously fit and well young adults. It highlights the importance of obtaining blood cultures prior to antibiotics in *all* patients admitted with possible sepsis, as this diagnosis may only be considered when *Fusobacterium necrophorum* is isolated from blood. Treatment involves prolonged antibiotics and drainage of abscesses. Prior to the advent of antibiotics the mortality was 30%–90%, but mortality is now estimated at between 5% and 17%.

Further Reading

 Bentham J, Pollard AJ, Milford CA, Anslow P, Pike MG. Cerebral infarct and meningitis secondary to Lemierre's syndrome. *Paediatr Neurol* 2004; **30**: 281–3.

Dalal A, Acharji S, Gehman M. Lemierre syndrome: forgotten but not extinct. *Infect Dis Clin Pract* 2007; **15**: 88–91.

deVeber G, Chan A, Monagle P *et al.* Anticoagulation therapy in pediatric patients with sinovenous thrombosis: a cohort study. *Arch Neurol* 1998; **55**: 1533–7.

Garcia J, Aboujaoude R, Apuzzio J, Alvarez JR. Septic pelvic thrombophlebitis: diagnosis and management. *Infect Dis Obstet Gynecol* 2006; 15614.

Hagelskjaer Kristensen L, Prag J. Human necrobacillosis, with emphasis on Lemierre's syndrome. *Clin Infect Dis* 2000; **31**: 524–32.

Hagelskjaer Kristensen L, Prag J. Lemierre's syndrome and other disseminated Fusobacterium necrophorum infections in Denmark: a prospective epidemiological and clinical survey. *Eur J Clin Microbiol Infect Dis* 2008; **27**: 779–89.

Hoehn KS. Lemierre's syndrome: the controversy of anticoagulation. *Pediatrics* 2005; **115**: 1415–16.

Lemierre A. On certain septicaemias due to anaerobic organisms. *Lancet* 1936; **227**: 701–3.

Levine SR, Twyman RE, Gilman E. The role of anticoagulation in cavernous sinus thrombosis. *Neurology* 1988; **38**: 517–22.

Riordan T. Human infection with *Fusobacterium necrophorum* (Necrobacillosis), with a focus on Lemierre's syndrome. *Clin Microbiol Rev* 2007; **20**: 622–59.

Sharma D, Rouphael N. Case report: atypical Lemierre's disease secondary to *Porphyromonas asaccharolytica*. *Curr Opin Pediatr* 2009; **21**: 397–400.

34 Leptospirosis

Emma Louise Hathorn

Case History

A 28-year-old man presented complaining of headache, myalgia, anorexia, fever and sweats. His symptoms had started approximately seven days after he had chased his dog into a marsh from which he had to be rescued. He smoked 20 cigarettes per day but was otherwise fit and well. The only significant findings on examination were tachycardia and bilateral conjunctival suffusion. Cerebrospinal fluid (CSF) examination showed 5 red blood cells, 507 white cells but no organisms. *Leptospira* immunoglobulin M (IgM) was negative from CSF but positive in serum at a titre of 1:640. Confirmatory direct microagglutination was positive at 1:160.

What is the differential diagnosis in this gentleman?

How would his doctor interpret his laboratory findings?

What are the treatment options for this gentleman?

Background

Leptospirosis is a zoonosis caused by the spiral-shaped Gram-negative spirochete, *Leptospira interrogans*. The genus *Leptospira*, belonging to the family Leptospiraceae, is divided into a number of species based on DNA hybridization. *L. interrogans* is the only species known to cause human disease. It is further classified serologically on the basis of variations in the lipopolysaccharide chains of its outer envelope. Human humoral immunity is directed at these chains and causes many of the clinical manifestations of leptospirosis.

Infected wild and domestic animals act as hosts, with leptospires persisting indefinitely in the convoluted tubules of the kidney prior to being shed in urine. Humans subsequently become infected when cuts, mucous membranes or conjunctivae come into contact, either with an infected animal, or water or soil contaminated by their urine. In this case, it is assumed that the patient was exposed to infected animal urine present in the marsh. Occupational exposures are more common, and these include veterinarians, abattoir workers, sewage workers and increasingly participants of water sports using inland waters.

The incubation period ranges from 2 to 30 days, with clinical symptoms typically presenting between days 5 to 14. Weil originally described a severe disease characterized by renal impairment and hepatitis with jaundice. Most commonly, however, it ranges from a subclinical disease detected by seroconversion to a mild self-limiting flu-like illness.

Symptomatic leptospirosis has two phases divided according to causative mechanism (Figure 34.1). The septicaemic phase is the result of a systemic vasculitis as leptospires multiply within the small blood vessel endothelium. There may be 1–3 days without fever after this, as specific IgM leptospiral antibodies are produced and leptospires disappear from the blood and CSF. This is followed by the immune phase during which lysis of leptospires results in extensive tissue damage. Approximately 50% report meningism. CSF analysis in this case was typical, demonstrating a reactive CSF with raised protein and lymphocytosis but no organism. As in the majority of cases, this patient recovered uneventfully and did not go on to develop any other organ involvement. It is not yet possible to identify the minority of patients who will develop severe disease at its onset.

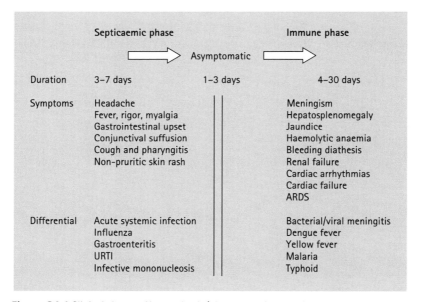

Figure 34.1 Clinical phases of leptospirosis (phases are often continuous and indistinct in severe disease). ARDS, acute respiratory distress syndrome; URTI, upper respiratory tract infection.

Isolation of leptospires remains the gold standard for the laboratory diagnosis of leptospirosis. Leptospires can be isolated from blood, CSF and urine during the first 7–10 days of the illness and from urine during the second and third weeks. The median time to detectable growth is 3 weeks but it can take up to 16 weeks. In clinical practice, serological diagnosis is therefore favoured.

A number of serological tests are available. In the case presented, an initial enzyme-linked immunosorbent assay (ELISA) screening test was used to detect the presence of IgM antibodies in both blood and CSF. Antibodies appear in the blood at detectable levels at about 5–10 days after the onset of disease. The result was then confirmed and identified to serovar level at the reference laboratory using the microscopic agglutination test. The test cannot distinguish between current, recent or past infection, and ideally two consecutive samples should be analysed looking for seroconversion or a fourfold increase in titre. The end-point of a single sample is highly debated but generally a titre of 1:800 is considered diagnostic with lower titres adding support to a compatible history or symptoms. False positives have been reported with syphilis, Lyme disease, legionellosis and relapsing fever.

The main consideration regarding treatment of this patient (Figure 34.2) is whether to commence antibiotics. A number of antibiotics including penicillins, tetracyclines, macrolides and chloramphenicol have been demonstrated to have antileptospiral activ-

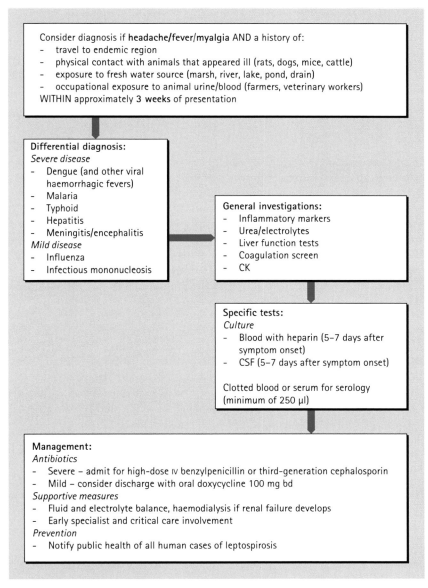

Consider diagnosis if **headache/fever/myalgia** AND a history of:
- travel to endemic region
- physical contact with animals that appeared ill (rats, dogs, mice, cattle)
- exposure to fresh water source (marsh, river, lake, pond, drain)
- occupational exposure to animal urine/blood (farmers, veterinary workers)

WITHIN approximately **3 weeks** of presentation

Differential diagnosis:
Severe disease
- Dengue (and other viral haemorrhagic fevers)
- Malaria
- Typhoid
- Hepatitis
- Meningitis/encephalitis

Mild disease
- Influenza
- Infectious mononucleosis

General investigations:
- Inflammatory markers
- Urea/electrolytes
- Liver function tests
- Coagulation screen
- CK

Specific tests:
Culture
- Blood with heparin (5–7 days after symptom onset)
- CSF (5–7 days after symptom onset)

Clotted blood or serum for serology (minimum of 250 µl)

Management:
Antibiotics
- Severe – admit for high-dose IV benzylpenicillin or third-generation cephalosporin
- Mild – consider discharge with oral doxycycline 100 mg bd

Supportive measures
- Fluid and electrolyte balance, haemodialysis if renal failure develops
- Early specialist and critical care involvement

Prevention
- Notify public health of all human cases of leptospirosis

Figure 34.2 Management algorithm for leptospirosis. CK, creatine kinase.

ity. Support for their use is controversial, however, and the evidence for their benefit and safety remains limited. In practice, however, it is generally accepted that symptomatic patients who present to medical services should receive antibiotic therapy: oral doxycycline for outpatients; and high-dose intravenous penicillins or a third-generation cephalosporin for severe disease requiring inpatient care. The patient presented was initially treated with ceftriaxone for suspected meningitis. This was later rationalized to intravenous benzylpenicillin. Concern regarding the safety of antibiotic use is largely due to reports of the Jarisch-Herxheimer reaction in cases where penicillin has been used.

Measures for the prevention of leptospirosis are generally targeted at the infected source (reducing animal reservoir populations; animal immunization; separation of animal and human habitations), transmission between source and human host (avoiding occupational and recreational sources of infection; dressing wounds) and infection in the host (increased awareness; doxycycline as post-exposure prophylaxis; vaccines). Human leptospirosis is a notifiable disease throughout the UK.

Recent Developments

Human vaccines derived from killed leptospires are currently in use in some countries including Japan and China. Efficacy rates are reported at 60%–100%. Their main disadvantage is that protective antibodies are only developed against the specific serovars present in the vaccine. The development of a cross-serovar vaccine is currently limited by a poor understanding of the mechanisms of both the pathogenicity and protective immunity of leptospirosis. Current work determining full genome sequences for individual serovars may allow the identification of genes encoding candidate vaccine proteins. Improved genetic analysis techniques may also allow the identification of virulence factors and subsequently enable risk stratification of patients at the onset of disease.

Conclusion

Leptospirosis is most commonly a subclinical disease that is self-limiting. Whilst antibiotics are widely available and known to have antileptospiral activity, their role remains controversial. It is difficult to be sure that they altered the clinical course or outcome in this patient. Leptospirosis is potentially fatal, however, and remains a diagnosis that should be considered in any patient with potential exposure.

Further Reading

Guidugli F, Castro AA, Atallah AN. Antibiotics for treating leptospirosis. *Cochrane Database Syst Rev* 2000; CD001306.

Koizumi N, Watanabe H. Leptospirosis vaccines: past, present, and future. *J Postgrad Med* 2005; **51**: 210–14.

Terpstra WJ. Human leptospirosis: guidance for diagnosis, surveillance and control. World Health Organization, 2003. Available at: http://www.who.int/csr/don/en/WHO_CDS_CSR_EPH_2002.23.pdf (accessed 12 08 11).

Infections in Special Circumstances

INFECTIONS IN CRITICAL CARE

PROBLEM

35 Ventilator-associated Pneumonia

Iain Gould, Vhairi M. Bateman

Case History

A 48-year-old man was admitted to hospital suffering from smoke inhalation following a house fire. His condition necessitated intubation and ventilation in the intensive care unit (ICU). He remained ventilated with an endotracheal tube 48 hours after his admission but subsequently developed pyrexia with purulent secretions noted from his chest on suction. Blood cultures were taken along with a bronchoalveolar lavage (BAL) sample. He was commenced on empirical treatment with tazobactam-piperacillin. The next day, blood cultures grew Gram-positive cocci in both bottles and the BAL specimen revealed growth of $>10^5$ colony-forming units/ml of *Staphylococcus aureus*. Linezolid was added to his antibiotic therapy pending further microbiology results. Two days after the onset of symptoms, ciprofloxacin-resistant methicillin-resistant *S. aureus* (MRSA) was confirmed from both blood cultures and the BAL specimen. The patient was moved to a side room and barrier nursing was commenced.

How is ventilator-associated pneumonia diagnosed?

What are the options for treating ventilator-associated pneumonia caused by MRSA?

Are there any potential strategies for preventing ventilator-associated pneumonia?

Background

Ventilator-associated pneumonia (VAP) is a common complication in ventilated patients and occurs in up to 27% of patients who require invasive ventilation. It is difficult to give precise figures regarding the mortality associated with VAP due to the number of confounding factors in critically ill patients, but estimates of mortality associated with VAP range from 20% to 50% and may be greater than 70% in those with infection due to multiresistant organisms. VAP also contributes significantly to morbidity, with increased ICU stay, prolonged need for mechanical ventilation and increased cost of hospitalization. The clinical features of VAP can be difficult to recognize. This makes the decision about when to start empirical antibiotic therapy difficult, especially as there is a need to limit the use of inappropriate antibiotics in order to slow the development of antibiotic resistance.

The clinical features of VAP include non-specific features of pyrexia and increased white blood cell count and C-reactive protein, but all of these may have an alternative explanation in the critically ill patient. More specific clinical features are purulent secretions on suction samples from the chest and increased need for respiratory support, and there may be chest X-ray changes. Chest X-rays in critically ill patients can be difficult to interpret since patients with VAP may have abnormal chest X-ray findings for other reasons, such as acute respiratory distress syndrome (ARDS) or pulmonary oedema. Patients with VAP seldom have the findings of a classic lobar pneumonia on chest X-ray.

Scoring systems have been proposed which aid the physician in making the diagnosis of VAP and instituting empirical antibiotic therapy when appropriate. The Clinical Pulmonary Infection Score (CPIS) is one such scoring system which has been validated for supporting the decision to institute empirical antibiotic therapy in patients with suspected VAP. A CPIS of greater than 6 is suggestive of infection. The scoring scheme is shown below in Box 35.1.

Box 35.1 The Clinical Pulmonary Infection Score (CPIS).

Clinical Pulmonary Infection Score (CPIS)

Temperature
- 0 point: 36.5–38.4°C
- 1 point: 38.5–38.9°C
- 2 points: <36 or >39°C

Blood leukocytes (cells/µl)
- 0 point: 4000–11 000
- 1 point: <4000 or >11 000
- 2 points: >500 band forms

Oxygenation (PaO$_2$/FiO$_2$)
- 0 point: PaO$_2$/FiO$_2$ >240 or ARDS
- 2 points: PaO$_2$/FiO$_2$ <240 and no evidence of ARDS

Pulmonary radiography
- 0 point: no infiltrate
- 1 point: diffuse or patchy infiltrates
- 2 points: localized infiltrate

Tracheal secretions (score)
- 0 point: <14
- 1 point: >14
- 2 points: purulent sputum

Culture of tracheal aspirate
- 0 point: minimal or no growth
- 1 point: moderate or more growth
- 2 points: moderate or greater growth

Total score of >6 points suggests ventilator-associated pneumonia.
ARDS, acute respiratory distress syndrome; FiO$_2$, inspired oxygen concentration; PaO$_2$, partial pressure of arterial oxygen.

The pathogenesis of VAP is most commonly associated with microaspiration of secretions from the oral cavity past the balloon of the endotracheal tube. The organisms in secretions can then set up infection in the lung tissue. Biofilms on the tracheal tube may also play a role. Haematogenous spread to the lung is relatively uncommon.

As well as microbiological factors there are a number of host factors which play an important role in the pathogenesis of VAP. Most ventilated patients are nursed lying supine which allows dependent secretions to build up in the lungs. Suction helps prevent the build-up of secretions within the lung but this does not eliminate microorganisms from the respiratory tract as effectively as coughing would in a non-ventilated patient. Additionally, lung tissue of ventilated patients is often abnormal. There may be coexistent ARDS, pulmonary oedema or pulmonary haemorrhage, all of which encourage microbial growth. Other risk factors for VAP include duration of mechanical ventilation, chronic pulmonary disease, neurological disease, trauma and red cell transfusions.

VAP is commonly associated with infection by Gram-negative bacilli such as *Pseudomonas aeruginosa*, *Klebsiella pneumoniae* and *Acinetobacter* spp. Patients within the ICU environment are also highly susceptible to colonization and infection with multi-resistant organisms. These include MRSA, multidrug-resistant *Pseudomonas*, *Serratia* spp., extended spectrum β-lactamase-producing *K. pneumoniae* and *Stenotrophomonas maltophilia*. The prevalence and predominance of these organisms vary widely between ICUs in different hospitals.

S. aureus can cause severe pneumonia. Several virulence mechanisms common to all *S. aureus* account for the severity of the pneumonia. Strains secreting the toxin Panton-Valentine leukocidin (PVL) can cause a severe form of necrotizing pneumonia associated with a poor prognosis. Currently, PVL-associated staphylococcal necrotizing pneumonia is predominantly a community-onset disease of adolescents and young adults.

Management options

The management options for MRSA VAP are either glycopeptides or linezolid. Glycopeptides, particularly vancomycin, are traditionally the mainstay of therapy. Vancomycin is safe and well tolerated and compares favourably to linezolid in terms of cost vs benefit.

Vancomycin therapy for MRSA VAP is associated with a 40% failure rate and there are some concerns regarding its use for this indication. Vancomycin therapy requires the measurement of serum drug levels to ensure that the dose being given is within the therapeutic range. It is primarily eliminated through the kidneys and patients with renal dysfunction require careful dosing with frequent measurement of serum drug levels. Patients in the ICU often have fluctuating levels of renal dysfunction, so achieving adequate dosing of vancomycin can be challenging. Physicians are more concerned about toxic rather than subtherapeutic doses but this may have contributed to the failure rate associated with vancomycin therapy. Previously, the recommended therapeutic range for vancomycin levels was trough levels of 5–10 mg/l. This has recently been increased to 10–20 mg/l with a recommendation for troughs of at least 15 mg/l in patients with severe MRSA infections. The pharmacokinetics of vancomycin show that it has a time-dependent bactericidal action and therefore the longer the serum concentration is maintained in the therapeutic range, the more efficacious vancomycin should be. To this end, vancomycin can be given as a continuous infusion rather than as twice-daily bolus doses, which allows the concentration of vancomycin in serum to be maintained. There is no consensus in the literature that this approach is superior to the twice-daily bolus dosing regimen and therefore vancomycin may be given by either method as long as it is monitored appropriately by serum trough levels. Under-dosing of vancomycin not only contributes to clinical failure but it may be associated with a trend for increasing minimum inhibitory concentrations (MICs) () of MRSA to vancomycin. Although absolute resistance to vancomycin (MIC >2 mg/l) remains rare, this MIC 'creep' tells us that MRSA is becoming tolerant to vancomycin. Coadministration of another drug along with the vancomycin, such as rifampicin or gentamicin, is often advocated with variable clinical effect.

Linezolid is an oxazolidinone antibiotic which targets the bacterial ribosome and has a bacteriostatic mechanism of action. Some studies have suggested that it is superior to vancomycin in the treatment of MRSA pneumonia since it reduces mortality. Additionally, linezolid has a toxin-suppressing effect in PVL-producing *S. aureus*. It can be combined with rifampicin in the management of PVL-associated MRSA pneumonia. A meta-analysis of the small subgroups of patients with MRSA bacteraemia enrolled in five trials comparing vancomycin and linezolid therapy showed no difference in outcome.

In this case, tazobactam-piperacillin was stopped and the patient improved with linezolid therapy. Ten days into his treatment he developed persistent hypertension which was thought to have been caused by linezolid, and the drug was stopped. He was weaned from the ventilator with the help of a tracheostomy and was discharged from the ICU by day 14. He remains colonized with MRSA at carrier sites and around the tracheostomy.

Comment

Empirical antibiotic therapy for VAP should be aimed at the most common causative pathogens, usually Gram-negative organisms, but will vary depending on the prevalent microorganisms within each ICU. The reason for starting linezolid as the first-line anti-staphylococcal treatment was that the patient had developed a severe pneumonia within 48 hours of admission to the ICU. As he was relatively young and thought to be in good health prior to admission, there was concern that the pneumonia may have been community acquired and therefore could have been community-associated *S. aureus*. Hypertension is a listed side effect of linezolid, although thrombocytopenia and neutropenia are more common. Optimum treatment of severe MRSA infections, excluding those with a deep source such as endocarditis and osteomyelitis, is usually 14 days of appropriate therapy. This is to prevent seeding of *S. aureus* to deep sites and/or metastatic complications.

Recent Developments

The most recently released anti-MRSA drugs to the market, daptomycin and tigecycline, are not recommended for the treatment of MRSA pneumonia. Daptomycin has been shown to be effective in the treatment of MRSA bacteraemia including endocarditis but it is inactivated by pulmonary surfactant and is contraindicated in the treatment of pneumonia. Tigecycline has demonstrated efficacy in complicated skin and soft tissue infection but has not yet been shown to be effective in the treatment of pneumonia. Caution may be required if considering using this drug as it has a very high tissue distribution and relatively low serum drug concentration, leading to concerns regarding its usefulness in patients with bacteraemia. Recent analysis of clinical trial data has suggested a relative increase in mortality in tigecycline-treated patients and perhaps this antibiotic should be avoided unless there are no other agents available.

Conclusion

Although there are controversies regarding the optimum treatment of MRSA VAP, there are perhaps greater controversies in the literature regarding the prevention of VAP.

Strategies to prevent VAP include using ventilator care bundles which are a combination of protocols. They include nursing the patient at an angle of 30–45°, daily sedation breaks, daily assessment for suitability of weaning the patient from the ventilator, peptic ulcer prophylaxis and deep vein thrombosis prophylaxis. Care bundles have been demonstrated to improve outcomes in ventilated patients, including a reduction in VAP. Other elements of preventing VAP include oral care and regular suction of secretions.

The most controversial strategy for preventing VAP is selective digestive tract decontamination (SDD). This is aimed at eradicating the normal oral flora which usually hosts the causative organisms of VAP. SDD includes topical antibiotics administered to the mouth, non-absorbable antibiotics and antifungals given by nasogastric tube and intravenous prophylactic antibiotics in some regimens. There have been conflicting studies in the literature, with some showing benefit from SDD and others no effect. There is concern that the effect of exposing patients to SDD will be to exert resistance pressure on the normal flora of patients in the ICU, increasing the acquisition of resistant organisms.

Further Reading

American Thoracic Society; Infectious Diseases Society of America. Guidelines for the management of adults with hospital-acquired, ventilator-associated, and healthcare-associated pneumonia. *Am J Respir Crit Care Med* 2005; **171**: 388–416.

Bonten MJM, Kollef MH, Hall JB. Risk factors for ventilator-associated pneumonia: from epidemiology to patient management. *Clin Infect Dis* 2004; **38**: 1141–9.

Cosgrove SE, Fowler VG Jr. Management of methicillin-resistant *Staphylococcus aureus* bacteremia. *Clin Infect Dis* 2008; **46**(Suppl 5): S386–93.

Rea-Neto A, Yousef NC, Tuche F *et al*. Diagnosis of ventilator-associated pneumonia: a systematic review of the literature. *Crit Care* 2008; **12**: R56.

Sakoulas G, Moellering RC Jr. Increasing antibiotic resistance among methicillin-resistant *Staphylococcus aureus* strains. *Clin Infect Dis* 2008; **46**(Suppl 5): S360–7.

Wunderink R, Rello J, Cammarata SK, Croos-Dabrera RV, Kollef MH. Linezolid vs vancomycin. analysis of two double-blind studies of patients with methicillin-resistant *Staphylococcus aureus* nosocomial pneumonia. *Chest* 2003; **124**: 1789–97.

PROBLEM

36 Pandemic Influenza A (H1N1) 2009

Kevin Rooney

Case History

A 32-year-old asthmatic, pregnant female at 24 weeks gestation presented to the antenatal clinic with a four-day history of fever, malaise, productive cough and worsening shortness of breath. On examination she was short of breath at rest, with a respiratory rate of 36 breaths/min, and was unable to speak in sentences. She had widespread inspiratory crackles with a saturation of peripheral oxygen (SpO$_2$) of 92% on high-flow oxygen therapy. Due to respiratory compromise, she was immediately transferred to the intensive care unit where she was sedated, intubated and mechanically ventilated. A diagnosis of an infective exacerbation of asthma was made and the patient was commenced on antiviral therapy, broad-spectrum antibiotics and standard medical therapy as per British Thoracic Society Guidelines on the management of asthma.

How do you make the diagnosis of pandemic influenza A (H1N1) 2009?

What constitutes severe disease in influenza (H1N1) 2009?

What are the risk factors for severe disease?

When should antiviral resistance be considered?

What other therapeutic options are available when mechanical ventilation fails?

Background

Pandemic influenza (H1N1) 2009 resulted in an unusual increase in the number of life-threatening respiratory infections and placed a major burden on intensive care services during 2009 and 2010/11. Clinicians are encouraged to diagnose H1N1 clinically on the basis of symptoms and to start antiviral treatment immediately prior to laboratory confirmation.

During the H1N1 pandemic, the clinical diagnostic criteria were fever (≥38°C) or a history of fever, and influenza-like illness (ILI; two or more of the following symptoms: cough, sore throat, rhinorrhoea, limb or joint pain, headache) or severe and/or life-threatening illness suggestive of an infective process. Other potential causes of the clinical presentation should be investigated and treated concurrently. Severe pandemic influenza infection should be suspected in any person with a history of recent ILI that progresses rapidly to severe medical illness (especially sepsis, pneumonia or exacerbation of underlying chronic illness) during a period when influenza is known to be circulating widely in the community. Severe disease can be defined as anyone with clinical and/

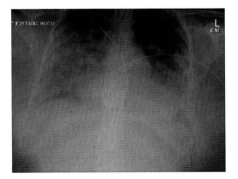

Figure 36.1 Chest X-ray demonstrating bilateral interstitial changes in H1N1 viral pneumonitis.

or radiological evidence of pneumonia (Figure 36.1), central nervous system signs and symptoms (altered mental status, seizures), shock and/or multiorgan failure, exacerbation of underlying disease and evidence of sustained virus replication or invasive secondary bacterial infection (e.g. persistent high fever and other symptoms beyond three days).

Although up to 50% of adults hospitalized with H1N1 were previously fit and healthy, risk factors identified for the development of complicated illness include: asthma and chronic obstructive pulmonary disease; morbid obesity; pregnancy and the immediate post-partum period; chronic cardiovascular, pulmonary, renal, hepatic or neurological conditions; diabetes mellitus; immunosuppression; and disadvantaged populations.

Warning signs of complicated illness include: dyspnoea and tachypnoea; hypoxia (oxygen pressure [pO_2] <8 kPa or SpO_2 <92%); hypercarbia; refractory hypotension and septic shock; acidosis; altered mental status; and persistent fever. Therefore, ward-based monitoring must include respiratory rate and pulse oximetry (SpO_2) on a regular basis.

Laboratory diagnosis

Respiratory tract specimens are recommended and nasopharyngeal samples may have the highest yield. In patients with lower respiratory tract symptoms, specimens from the lower respiratory tract (tracheal and bronchial aspirates) have a higher diagnostic yield. Reverse transcriptase–polymerase chain reaction (RT-PCR) is the diagnostic method of choice for pandemic influenza (H1N1) 2009. It detects the presence of the virus RNA and can distinguish pandemic influenza (H1N1) 2009 from other influenza virus subtypes. RT-PCR has both a high sensitivity (86%–100%) and high specificity for the diagnosis of pandemic influenza (H1N1) 2009.

Rapid influenza diagnostic tests are not generally very useful in initial individual patient management as the test sensitivity is variable and may miss pandemic (H1N1) virus infection. The results of all influenza diagnostic tests are dependent upon several factors including specimen type, quality of specimen collection, timing of collection, and storage and transport conditions. All of these factors may result in false-negative results. When the clinical suspicion of pandemic (H1N1) 2009 infection is high, then clinicians should consider repeat testing if initial tests are negative. In a setting of high clinical suspicion, treatment and infection control measures for pandemic influenza (H1N1) should not be withdrawn following a negative result.

Treatment and infection control

Oseltamivir is the first-line antiviral agent for H1N1, including for the treatment of pregnant women. Early treatment is associated with best outcome but improvements may still be seen even when treatment is commenced beyond the first 48 hours of illness. Before a patient's influenza status is known they should be nursed in isolation where possible. Confirmed cases can be nursed in open, cohorted areas if side rooms are unavailable. Infection control measures can be discontinued 24 hours after symptom resolution, unless the patient is thought to be at risk of prolonged virus excretion or oseltamivir resistance (e.g. immunocompromised patients), and timely hospital discharge is preferred.

Oseltamivir resistance is uncommon in influenza (H1N1) 2009 but should be considered in patients with persistence of fever after five days of therapy and in severely immunocompromised individuals. Intravenous zanamivir may be considered on a compassionate-use basis when oseltamivir resistance is known or suspected. Inhaled zanamivir is not recommended in critically ill patients as it is not systemically active.

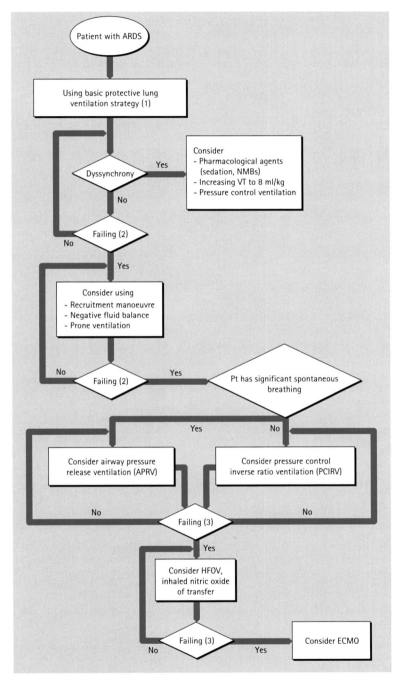

Figure 36.2 An example of an advanced mechanical ventilation algorithm from the Royal Alexandra Hospital, Paisley. ARDS, acute respiratory distress syndrome; ECMO, extracorporeal membrane oxygenation; HFOV, high-frequency oscillatory ventilation; NMB, neuromuscular blocking agent; Pt, patient; VT, tidal volume.

Up to 25% of ventilated cases have a concurrent bacterial infection. *Streptococcus pneumoniae*, group A *Streptococcus* and *Staphylococcus aureus* have all been isolated from patients diagnosed with influenza. Local guidelines for the investigation and antibiotic treatment of community-acquired pneumonia should be followed.

Recent Developments

There is no evidence to support the use of high-dose steroids in the treatment of pandemic influenza (H1N1). In H5N1 (avian flu), high-dose steroids worsened outcome and increased viral shedding times.

The ventilatory management of cases of pandemic influenza (H1N1) is complex and should follow an advanced mechanical ventilation strategy incorporating protective lung ventilation and a significantly negative fluid balance (Figure 36.2).

Conclusion

H1N1 infection requiring ventilation poses significant challenges to clinicians, and mortality is high despite advanced mechanical ventilation strategies. As in other reversible pulmonary complications requiring ventilation, consideration should be given to early referral for extracorporeal membrane oxygenation (ECMO) in cases of refractory hypoxaemia. The current referral criteria for ECMO in the UK are a ratio of partial pressure of arterial oxygen:inspired oxygen concentration (PaO_2/FiO_2 ratio) <10 and less than seven days of:

- High inspired oxygen requirements (FiO_2 >0.8)
- High peak inspiratory pressures >30 cmH$_2$O

Further Reading

Australia and New Zealand Extracorporeal Membrane Oxygenation (ANZ ECMO) Influenza Investigators, Davies A, Jones D, Bailey M *et al*. Extracorporeal Membrane Oxygenation for 2009 Influenza A (H1N1) Acute Respiratory Distress Syndrome. *JAMA* 2009; **302**: 1888–95.

Hui DS, Lee N, Chan PK. Clinical management of pandemic 2009 influenza A (H1N1) infection. *Chest* 2010; **137**: 916–25.

Lim WS, Baudouin SV, George RC *et al*. BTS guidelines for the management of community acquired pneumonia in adults: update 2009. *Thorax* 2009; **64**(Suppl 3): iii1–55.

Napolitano LM, Park PK, Raghavendran K, Bartlett RH. Nonventilatory strategies for patients with life-threatening 2009 H1N1 influenza and severe respiratory failure. *Crit Care Med* 2010; **38**(4 Suppl): e74–90.

WHO guidelines for pharmacological management of pandemic (H1N1) 2009 influenza and other influenza viruses. World Health Organization, 2010. Available at: http://www.who.int/csr/resources/publications/swineflu/h1n1_use_antivirals_20090820/en/index.html (accessed 13 09 11).

Writing Committee of the WHO Consultation on Clinical Aspects of Pandemic (H1N1) 2009 Influenza, Bautista E, Chotpitayasunondh T, Gao Z *et al*. Clinical aspects of pandemic 2009 influenza A (H1N1) virus infection. *N Engl J Med* 2010; **362**: 1708–19.

37 Intensive Care Unit Sepsis in Multiorgan Failure

Andrew Berrington

Case History

A 34-year-old woman was admitted with pneumonia and required ventilation on the intensive care unit. She was treated initially with intravenous cefuroxime and erythromycin but was switched to benzylpenicillin when blood cultures grew *Streptococcus pneumoniae*. Despite this treatment she continued to mount a vigorous inflammatory response with fever, tachycardia and a high neutrophil count. Five days after admission she was in established multiorgan failure, ventilated, on inotropes and requiring haemodialysis. The medical consultant visited the intensive care unit, crossed off the penicillin and prescribed meropenem plus piperacillin-tazobactam.

What is the likely cause of her ongoing illness?

Is this change of antibiotics sensible?

What else could be done for this patient?

Background

This previously well patient was admitted with severe community-acquired pneumonia (CAP). Blood cultures confirmed the aetiology to be a penicillin-susceptible strain of *Streptococcus pneumoniae*, which permitted a switch from cefuroxime plus erythromycin (which is a standard catch-all treatment for CAP) to penicillin; this incidentally illustrates the importance of taking blood cultures from patients with pneumonia. Penicillin has a narrower spectrum, which should reduce the risk of antibiotic-related complications such as acquisition of resistant flora or *Clostridium difficile* infection, and is arguably more potent than cefuroxime against susceptible strains. Some people believe that pneumococcal bacteraemia responds better to β-lactam/macrolide combinations than to β-lactam agents alone, but this is controversial and penicillin monotherapy in adequate doses is reasonable treatment.

Why then does the patient remain so unwell? Perhaps because she has developed septic shock, which can sustain itself even after the infective trigger has been dealt with. Sepsis and related terms are often misused but it is important to understand their proper meanings. Sepsis is defined as a systemic inflammatory response syndrome (SIRS) associated with suspected or proven infection. SIRS can be defined as the systemic manifestations of infection, which can be variable, but a practical definition is to require at least two of: abnormal core temperature (<36°C or >38.3°C); tachycardia (heart rate >90 beats/min); tachypnoea (respiratory rate >20 breaths/min); and an abnormal white blood cell count (<4 or >12 × 10⁹/l). If sepsis is complicated by organ dysfunction (for instance renal or respiratory failure) it is called severe sepsis, and if hypotension persists despite adequate fluid resuscitation it is called septic shock (Figure 37.1).

Sepsis represents interdependent physiological cascades that depend on both the host and the infecting organism. Sepsis is initiated by the interaction between cells of the innate immune system and molecules such as lipopolysaccharide expressed by the infecting organism. This leads to an increase in production of cytokines such as tumour necrosis factor, interleukin-1, interleukin-6 and platelet-activating factor, which as well as helping to recruit the adaptive immune response, also activate the coagulation cascade and cause direct and indirect injury, particularly to endothelial cells. The synthesis of nitric oxide, a potent vasodilator, is also upregulated. If these responses overwhelm their natural control mechanisms they can become detrimental instead of helpful, and the result is a syndrome of illness characterized by vasodilatation, capillary leakage, disseminated intravascular coagulation and variable end-organ damage particularly affecting the heart, lungs and kidneys. Once initiated, patients can remain septic even after control of the initiating infection has been achieved, a situation which might be partly but not completely explained by persistence of bacterial antigens.

The patient described has septic shock and is surviving only because she is receiving full supportive care. The medical consultant under whom she was admitted visits the intensive care unit and is concerned over her condition. The consultant does not think that penicillin is a sufficiently powerful antibiotic so a combination of meropenem and piperacillin-tazobactam is subsequently prescribed. Although well meant, this is not sensible. The working diagnosis is septic shock, which although initiated by pneumococcal infection can be both persistent and severe despite elimination of the initiating infection. It is sometimes the case that laboratory results do not translate into a clinical response, but at this point antibiotic failure is unlikely to be the cause of her condition. Furthermore, the consultant's concept of 'switching to more powerful antibiotics' is flawed: the pharmacodynamics of penicillin against pneumococci in the blood or lungs are likely to be at least as good as those of either meropenem or piperacillin-tazobactam, and moreover there is no reason why two β-lactam drugs in combination should be better than one. This consultant is probably making the common error of confusing spectrum with potency. There is also a more general point that intensive care units should not allow visiting clinicians to change therapy without the agreement of the intensivists; this should apply to the drug chart just as much as inotrope dosing or ventilator settings.

The patient is quickly switched back to penicillin in a dose appropriate to her renal support, but antibiotics, while important, are only one of several therapies necessary. Sepsis requires 'goal-directed therapy' (i.e. the maintenance of physiological parameters as close to normal as possible), which is achieved by: management on an intensive care unit with respiratory support, renal replacement, inotropic drugs and careful fluid management; ventilation that does not damage the lungs (usually achieved by using low tidal volumes); and appropriate anti-infectives. In this case the antibiotics were directed against *S. pneumoniae* but where the aetiology is unknown it can be necessary to use broader-spectrum agents. In some cases the inflammatory cascade can be modified using activated protein C, which is discussed later. The use of steroids in sepsis is controversial

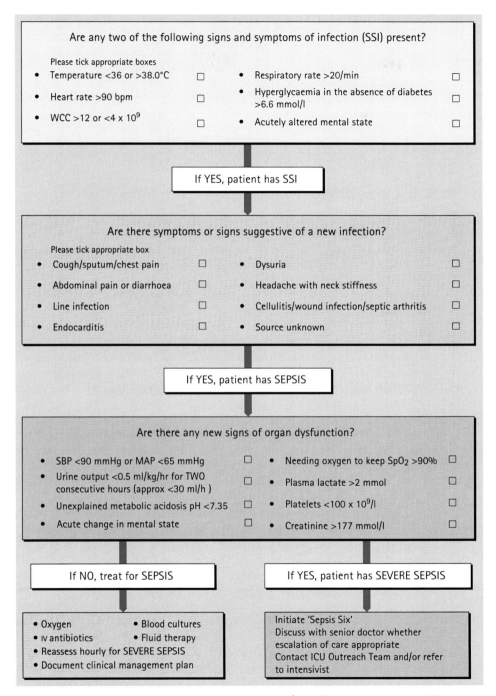

Figure 37.1 Diagnosis and management of sepsis. bpm, beats/min; ICU, intensive care unit; MAP, mean arterial pressure; SBP, systolic blood pressure; SpO$_2$, oxygen saturation; WCC, white blood cell count.

– current consensus is that high-dose steroids aimed at modulating the immune system are not beneficial, but that low-dose steroids aimed at replacing physiological deficits might be. Ventilated patients on intensive care units are also vulnerable to numerous complications that should be actively prevented. Pressure-area care is hugely important, physiotherapy is thought to be helpful in preventing contractures, nutritional needs must be attended to, and the risk of secondary infection must be minimized, for instance through care of vascular access lines, urinary catheters and the airway.

Despite optimal management, septic shock has a high mortality, and unfortunately the patient described died eight days after admission.

Recent Developments

The Surviving Sepsis Campaign (SSC) is an international collaboration, established in 2002, aimed at improving outcomes in severe sepsis and specifically at reducing the relative mortality by 25% by 2009. Guidelines for managing sepsis have been produced under the SSC banner and were updated in 2008. Among comprehensive recommendations these emphasize early goal-directed resuscitation (to maintain arterial and venous pressure, urine output and oxygenation at appropriate levels) combined with early administration of appropriate antibiotics plus any other measures such as surgery that are indicated to control the infective source. It is now firmly established that the earlier patients receive appropriate antimicrobials, the better the outcome, which means that treatment should be discussed with an expert and initiated as soon as possible rather than, for instance, left until the next drug round. In the UK these guidelines are supported by formalized care bundles, one of which incorporates the 'sepsis six' concept, referring to six simple tasks that should be performed within the first hour of a case of sepsis being recognized. These are administration of 100% oxygen, taking blood cultures, administration of intravenous antibiotics, starting fluid resuscitation, checking the haemoglobin and lactate, and placing and monitoring a urinary catheter. It is in the initial recognition and management of sepsis that the greatest gains can be made, and these ideas are now actively promoted by intensive care departments to non-specialist areas.

Manipulation of the inflammatory mediators involved in sepsis has long been proposed as a therapeutic modality, but laboratory studies have proved difficult to translate into clinical advances. High-dose steroids, antibodies against endotoxin, tumour necrosis factor antagonists and interleukin-1 receptor antagonists, all of which showed promise in animal models, have failed in clinical trials. However, administration of recombinant human activated protein C (whose naturally occurring counterpart is abnormally reduced in sepsis) has been shown to improve the outcome of severe sepsis in adult patients who, on clinical grounds, are deemed at high risk of death. It is given by infusion over 96 hours and is proposed to have several effects on host inflammatory and procoagulant responses (which are closely linked), generally promoting fibrinolysis and inhibiting thrombosis and inflammation. It is not a magic bullet: 16 patients need to be treated in order to save one life, and it has a high incidence of side effects such as bleeding. Furthermore, more recent trials have failed to confirm that it is genuinely beneficial.

Although it was obvious in the case described, in less severe cases it can be difficult to distinguish between sepsis (SIRS caused by infection) and non-infective SIRS. Serum markers such as C-reactive protein are unhelpful here because they can be elevated in all inflammatory conditions, both infective and non-infective. A serum marker called procalcitonin has been proposed to be more specific for infection, particularly bacterial infection, but its early promise has not been entirely borne out.

Septic patients on the intensive care unit are at risk of secondary infections, particularly ventilator-associated pneumonia. There is much debate about the place of selective digestive tract decontamination (SDD), whereby a combination of systemic and topical antibiotics is given to reduce bacterial populations in the gut with the aim of reducing the risk of pneumonia. There is reasonable evidence in favour of this practice but it is often resisted because of fears of antibiotic resistance and side effects, and it is true that the studies that found its benefits to exceed its risks were performed before the emergence of challenges such as extended spectrum β-lactamases and hypervirulent *Clostridium difficile*. Currently we have guidelines that recommend SDD and others (including guidance from the National Institute for Health and Clinical Excellence that is binding for National Health Service hospitals) that do not. There are repeated calls for SDD to be investigated again in a current, UK setting, but for now the question is likely to remain unanswered. Finally, there is also limited evidence in favour of giving nebulized prophylactic antibiotics such as colistin, again to reduce the risk of ventilator-associated pneumonia.

Conclusion

Sepsis, and particularly severe sepsis and septic shock, carry a high mortality and merit vigorous and expert treatment. It is important to treat the initiating infection appropriately and early, but antimicrobials are just one among a variety of therapeutic strategies that must be optimized, preferably on an intensive care unit. Experience with immunomodulatory drugs has been disappointing, but further advances in our understanding of this complex condition may reveal new opportunities for intervention.

Further Reading

Bernard GR, Vincent JL, Laterre PF *et al*. Efficacy and safety of recombinant human activated protein C for severe sepsis. *N Engl J Med* 2001; **344**: 699–709.

Dellinger RP, Levy MM, Carlet JM *et al*. Surviving Sepsis Campaign: international guidelines for management of severe sepsis and septic shock: 2008. *Intensive Care Med* 2008; **34**: 17–60.

Lever A, Mackenzie I. Sepsis: definition, epidemiology, and diagnosis. *BMJ* 2007; **335**: 879–83.

Mackenzie I, Lever A. Management of sepsis. *BMJ* 2007; **335**: 929–32.

National Institute for Health and Clinical Excellence. Technical patient safety solutions for ventilator-associated pneumonia in adults (PSG002). NICE, 2008. Available at: http://guidance.nice.org.uk/PSG002 (accessed 05 09 11).

Russell JA. Management of sepsis. *N Engl J Med* 2006; **355**: 1699–713.

Tang BMP, Eslick GD, Craig JC, McLean AS. Accuracy of procalcitonin for sepsis diagnosis in critically ill patients: systematic review and meta-analysis. *Lancet Infect Dis* 2007; **7**: 210–17.

38 Candidaemia

Thomas Patterson

Case History

A 23-year-old man who was previously healthy was admitted to the surgical intensive care unit (ICU) following a gunshot wound to the abdomen. Exploratory laparotomy revealed a perforated colon which required a temporary diverting colonostomy. He was now post-operative day ten with a complicated course that included total parenteral nutrition through a right subclavian catheter. He remained intubated with persistent fever and sepsis, with hypotension, an elevated serum creatinine, and leukocytosis, despite antibiotic therapy with piperacillin-tazobactam. Urine cultures taken two days prior were positive for a *Candida* species other than *C. albicans*, with a final identification pending. Blood cultures were now positive for an unidentified 'yeast'.

How would you manage the patient at this point?

Should additional tests or procedures be performed?

What are the best therapeutic options for this patient?

Background

Candidaemia is a leading cause of nosocomial bloodstream infection worldwide with associated attributable mortality rates in most series around 40%. These infections have a significant impact on medical costs and prolonged hospital stay. Thus, it is imperative to understand the epidemiology, pathogenesis, risk factors and management strategies to improve outcomes in critically ill patients at risk for these infections. Infections due to *Candida* species can range from asymptomatic colonization or mucosal infection to uncomplicated candidaemia to that of deep-seated or end-organ infection (e.g. abscesses, endophthalmitis, chronic disseminated candidiasis of the liver and spleen, and others). The presentation is determined in part by underlying risk or host factors.

In many institutions, the epidemiology of *Candida* infection has shifted from that of *Candida albicans*, which is considered the most pathogenic species but is responsible for less than half of the invasive isolates in most centres worldwide, to that of *C. glabrata, C. parapsilosis, C. tropicalis, C. krusei*, and others. This shift in epidemiology is important as many of these non-*C. albicans* strains (especially *C. glabrata* and *C. krusei*) are resistant to fluconazole. Others occur in specific epidemiological settings. For example, *C. parapsilosis* is particularly common in neonates and associated with catheter infections – and is a species very difficult to eradicate without catheter removal. It is important to realize as well that these non-*C. albicans* organisms are more likely to occur in the setting of prior azole therapy or prophylaxis, which must be considered in selecting empirical antifungal therapy.

In this patient, risk factors for invasive candidiasis included prior antibiotic therapy, a central venous catheter, total parenteral nutrition, surgery which involved transection of the gut wall, colonization of the urinary tract with yeast, and critical illness. Other identified risk factors for invasive candidiasis include immunosuppression, comorbid illnesses (diabetes, malignancy, pancreatitis, etc.), length of stay in the ICU and others. Several prediction rules for assessing likelihood of infection have been developed, ranging from a relatively simple 'colonization index' to more elaborate prediction rules based on inclusion of more risk characteristics. While these can be helpful, especially in clinical trial settings, as a clinician the important lesson is that the diagnosis of invasive candidiasis must be considered in patients with these risk factors and that cultures of blood and other body fluids are taken not only to establish a culture-based diagnosis of invasive candidiasis but also to evaluate for the presence or absence of other infections as well.

The benefit of early treatment of candidaemia has been evaluated in a number of settings. In several studies, the early institution of antifungal therapy has been associated with significantly decreased in-hospital mortality. While antifungal therapy beginning within 24 hours of the culture being drawn is associated with improved outcomes, it should be realized that even with newer blood culture technology, cultures may take more than 30 hours on average to turn positive. Thus, strong suspicion of infection and lack of other documented causes should lead to consideration of early, pre-emptive initiation of antifungal therapy.

Guidelines have been recently published incorporating new treatment recommendations. Fluconazole has been a mainstay for treating candidaemia based on clinical trial data and extensive experience. While the agent is extremely well tolerated and effective and is now inexpensive, the shift to less susceptible species raises concerns about treatment failures, especially before susceptibility results are known or in seriously ill patients. This is especially true for some species of yeast such as *C. glabrata*, which may develop resistance to fluconazole or cause breakthrough infection, or *C. krusei* which is intrinsically resistant to fluconazole. Thus, the echinocandins have become the recommended therapy, especially in critically ill patients, in those with neutropenia and in patients with prior azole therapy or those species of *Candida* previously mentioned. There are minimal clinical differences between echinocandins identified to this point and differential susceptibility between the agents for resistant strains is also limited. These agents are only given intravenously but are rapidly fungicidal for most *Candida* species with the notable exception of *C. parapsilosis* which has elevated minimum inhibitory concentrations for all the available echinocandins.

The concept of step-down therapy following an initial course of intravenous therapy with an echinocandin is strongly encouraged, although the timing of this is supported by limited data. Fluconazole is particularly useful in this regard, although voriconazole is also effective for isolates or species resistant to fluconazole.

Recommended management

In this patient, early therapy with an echinocandin is strongly recommended, pending confirmation of the species identification. The presence of a yeast other than *C. albicans* in the urine suggests that the organism in blood will be another species as well. While urinary concentrations of the echinocandins are minimal, the urine culture is used in this setting more as a clue to unidentified invasive infection than as a urinary tract infection *per se*. Similarly, if the sputum were positive for yeasts, it would be unlikely to indicate true pneumonia but rather reflect colonization and serve as a risk factor for invasive infection.

It is very important to identify the species of *Candida* as it can serve as a surrogate for likely susceptibility, as patterns of antifungal susceptibility are predictable based on species alone. On the other hand, it is reasonable to test most *Candida* isolates from blood or other sterile sites for antifungal susceptibility, which can be useful in guiding additional antifungal therapy including specific choices for step-down therapy.

An area of recent controversy is that of line removal. While it is difficult to show that central catheter line removal definitively results in improved outcomes in all patients, fungaemia can be prolonged with the catheter in place, particularly in ICU patients in whom the catheter is a likely portal of entry. In other patients with long-term tunnelled catheters, especially patients with haematological malignancy and mucositis, a gastrointestinal site is a likely source of infection and line removal may not facilitate clearance of the organism. However, some species, like *C. parapsilosis*, are extremely difficult to eliminate without line removal, such that line removal is usually recommended in patients with that organism.

This patient was empirically treated with an echinocandin, and the organism in urine and blood was identified as *C. glabrata*. The organism was tested and found to be susceptible to fluconazole. The line was removed and subsequent blood cultures were negative. No evidence of endophthalmitis was found. The patient was changed to oral fluconazole as his gut function had improved and he completed a 14-day course of antifungal therapy.

Recent Developments

Extensive efforts have aimed at improving the early diagnosis of invasive candidiasis. Scoring systems have been refined which identify high-risk patients who may benefit from early pre-emptive therapy or even prophylaxis. Efforts to provide more prompt identification of yeast species have been introduced including peptide–nucleic acid systems, which can rapidly identify certain *Candida* species, and the use of chromogenic agar which can also provide relatively rapid species identification. Non-culture-based assays – such as the detection of fungal cell wall 1,3-β-D-glucan (which is not specific for *Candida* but may be an early indication of invasive infection), other cell-wall antigens, or molecular targets – are aimed at further improving the diagnosis of invasive *Candida* infections.

Conclusion

1   In patients at high risk for invasive candidiasis, prompt diagnosis and therapy are essential to a successful outcome.

2   Risk factors for invasive candidiasis include broad-spectrum antibiotic use, central venous catheterization, total parenteral nutrition, ICU stay, gastrointestinal tract

surgery, urinary tract colonization with *Candida*, immunosuppression and other comorbidity (malignancy and diabetes).

3   Blood and other body fluids should be cultured to establish the diagnosis of invasive candidiasis.

4   Consider empirical antifungal therapy in the setting of persistent unexplained fever and leukocytosis in a patient in the ICU/high-dependency unit, especially in the presence of other risk factors for candidaemia including positive *Candida* cultures from other sites.

5   Use an echinocandin for unstable patients with moderate to severe infection, for patients with neutropenia, and in the setting of prior azole use. Fluconazole can be considered for stable, non-neutropenic patients with less severe disease.

6   Antifungal therapy should be continued for a minimum of 14 days after the last positive blood culture.

7   Oral step-down therapy based on identification and susceptibility of the organism is strongly encouraged.

8   Clinical performance measures include:
    1   Starting therapy within 24 hours of a positive culture.
    2   Obtaining a dilated eye examination to exclude candidal ophthalmitis.
    3   Obtaining follow-up blood cultures to document clearance of the organism.

Further Reading

Brass EP, Edwards JE. Should the guidelines for management of central venous catheters in patients with candidemia be changed now? *Clin Infect Dis* 2010; **51**: 304–6.

Mohr JF, Sims C, Paetznick V *et al.* Prospective survey of (1,3)-beta-D-glucan and its relationship to invasive candidiasis in the surgical intensive care unit setting. *J Clin Microbiol* 2011; **49**: 58–61.

Morrell M, Fraser VJ, Kollef MH. Delaying the empiric treatment of *Candida* bloodstream infection until positive blood culture results are obtained: a potential risk factor for hospital mortality. *Antimicrob Agents Chemother* 2005; **49**: 3640–5.

Ostrosky-Zeichner L, Kullberg BJ, Bow EJ *et al.* Early treatment of candidemia in adults: a review. *Med Mycol* 2011; **49**: 113–20.

Ostrosky-Zeichner L, Pappas PG. Invasive candidiasis in the intensive care unit. *Crit Care Med* 2006; **34**: 857–63.

Pappas PG, Kauffman CA, Andes D *et al.* Clinical practice guidelines for the management of candidiasis: 2009 update by the Infectious Diseases Society of America. *Clin Infect Dis* 2009; **48**: 503–35.

IMMUNOCOMPROMISED PATIENT

PROBLEM

39 Invasive Aspergillosis

Thomas Patterson

Case History

A 45-year-old man with acute myelogenous leukaemia which was refractory to chemotherapy had undergone allogeneic haematopoietic stem cell transplant two months prior to his presentation with fever and shortness of breath. His course was complicated by graft-versus-host disease requiring high-dose corticosteroid therapy. He was receiving fluconazole antifungal prophylaxis. Examination revealed a temperature of 39°C, respiratory rate of 22 breaths/min and bilateral crackles on lung auscultation. Evaluation included a chest computed tomography (CT) scan which showed a nodular lesion in the right lower lobe surrounded by a zone of low attenuation; peripheral white blood cell count was 0.2×10^9/l and a platelet count was 82×10^9/l. Blood cultures were drawn and a serum galactomannan test was ordered, and he was started on broad-spectrum antibacterial therapy empirically with cefepime and vancomycin.

How would you manage the patient at this point?

What is your suspicion for invasive aspergillosis?

Should additional evaluation be performed?

What are the best therapeutic options for this patient?

Background

Invasive fungal infections are a major cause of morbidity and mortality in severely ill patients with haematological malignancy and in those undergoing marrow and stem cell transplantation. In these patients careful consideration of risk factors is important in assessing likelihood of an invasive fungal infection, as the risk for infection due to invasive moulds is extremely high. Factors which predict increased risk of invasive fungal infection include prolonged neutropenia, the use of high doses of corticosteroid therapy, cytotoxic chemotherapy, solid organ or haematopoietic stem cell transplantation, and the development of graft-versus-host disease, among others. Even among patients with similar underlying diseases, risk can vary dramatically depending on factors such as status of underlying malignancy, response to chemotherapy and the timing of infection. For example, in patients with acute leukaemia, risk will be dramatically higher in those with relapse of underlying disease or in those who are refractory to chemotherapy than in those with initial induction therapy, which compares to an even lower risk in those receiving consolidation or maintenance therapy after an initial favourable response to chemotherapy. Similarly, repeated use of immunosuppressive agents including corticosteroids or extended periods with neutrophil deficiency will further increase risk. Thus, in this patient, strong consideration should be given to the possible diagnosis of an invasive fungal infection, particularly in the setting of secondary neutropenia associated with graft-versus-host disease and with the clinical presentation of pulmonary symptoms.

In patients with haematological malignancy and in those patients undergoing stem cell transplantation, invasive moulds are more likely than infection due to yeasts, particularly in the setting of fluconazole prophylaxis. While concerns have been raised regarding the emergence of *Mucorales* species and the occurrence of other resistant moulds, like *Fusarium* and Scedosporium species, invasive *Aspergillus* is the most common mould that should be considered in this setting. However, because specific therapy can be targeted to some of these pathogens (like agents of mucormycosis which are resistant to voriconazole but susceptible to polyene therapy), the establishment of a microbiological diagnosis is crucial to successful management of these patients.

Therapy is more likely to be successful if begun promptly and if the underlying causes of immunosuppression resolve – such as recovery from neutropenia or successful transplantation or response to chemotherapy. However, the diagnosis of infection is difficult to establish as cultures of blood and other body fluids in invasive aspergillosis are often negative, even with more advanced infection. Non-culture-based diagnostics have been extensively investigated for *Aspergillus*. Currently, biomarkers that measure cell wall galactomannan (Platelia *Aspergillus*, Sanofi Diagnostics Pasteur, Marnes-la-Coquette, France; Bio-Rad, Redmond, WA, USA) and detect $1,3$-β-D-glucan using a *Limulus* lysate-based assay (Fungitell, Associates of Cape Cod, Falmouth, MA, USA) are commercially available. The sensitivity of galactomannan detection is significantly reduced by a number of factors including anti-mould active therapy or prophylaxis, a limited number of samples and others. In addition, false-positive results may occur in the setting of administration of some antibiotics, most notably piperacillin-tazobactam, in neonates, and in some dietary sources. Polymerase chain reaction-based molecular assays are still investigational but show promise for diagnosis. All these assays are likely to be even more sensitive when testing on bronchoalveolar lavage fluid but performance of the assays in those settings is less extensively studied.

Radiological findings are also very helpful in suggesting a likely diagnosis of infection. Classically, a nodular lesion surrounded by a 'halo' of ground glass attenuation is associated with invasive aspergillosis. Although not diagnostic (nodular lesions with a halo sign can occur in bacterial infections as well as infections due to other fungi), in high-risk patients it is associated with invasive aspergillosis and can spur an attempt at a microbiological diagnosis along with consideration for empirical antifungal therapy while an evaluation is being performed (Figure 39.1). The absence of a halo should not dissuade the diagnosis, as these signs are often fleeting. On the other hand, the absence of a nodular lesion makes the diagnosis less likely, as nodular lesions have usually been seen in most patients with invasive pulmonary aspergillosis in clinical trials. These pulmonary nodules will often cavitate, which occurs later in the course of infection and is, in fact, often a more favourable sign as it correlates with recovery of neutrophils.

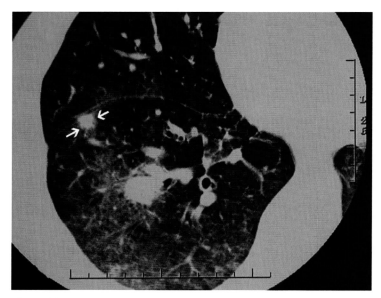

Figure 39.1 CT scan showing the classic nodular lesion surrounded by a 'halo' of ground glass attenuation (arrows) associated with invasive aspergillosis.

Voriconazole is the recommended therapy in most patients with invasive aspergillosis, based on a large global trial with superior outcomes and better survival compared to amphotericin B deoxycholate. Voriconazole offers the advantage of intravenous as well as oral therapy options, and it has been reasonably well tolerated. Nevertheless, there are a number of important considerations including drug interactions, lack of activity against *Mucorales* spp., limited use of the intravenous formulation in renal insufficiency, and adverse reactions (especially hepatic toxicity and rash, along with the well-described visual toxicities, although the latter is unlikely to be serious or dose limiting). Thus, liposomal amphotericin B is recommended as an alternative primary agent in some patients, especially in those in whom voriconazole is contraindicated or cannot be tolerated. Measurement of voriconazole levels should be considered especially in those on oral therapy. Initial combination therapy is not recommended in most patients but is an area undergoing active clinical investigation.

Recommended management

In this patient, prompt consideration of risk and an attempt to establish a diagnosis are important in successful management. Empirical therapy in high-risk patients *while a diagnostic evaluation is being conducted* is recommended based on clinical suspicion of an invasive fungal infection. In this patient, empirical broad-spectrum antibiotics are indicated based on fever and neutropenia. Pulmonary symptoms strongly suggest the presence of a pulmonary pathogen but, even in their absence, CT of the chest is indicated due to lack of sensitivity of a chest radiograph. Non-culture-based diagnostics based on availability (usually a serum galactomannan) are indicated. Consideration for a bronchoalveolar lavage (BAL) should be promptly undertaken to increase the likelihood of establishing a diagnosis – cultures, cytology and BAL galactomannan are all possible means to establish a diagnosis. Voriconazole would be the recommended empirical antifungal agent in this patient. If the patient had previously received voriconazole, then a broadened differential including *Mucorales* spp. would suggest the empirical use of liposomal amphotericin B.

This patient was initially begun on voriconazole 6 mg/kg twice daily for two doses, followed by 4 mg/kg intravenously twice daily. He underwent bronchoscopy which showed fungal elements consistent with a hyaline mould and cultures confirmed *Aspergillus flavus*. He responded clinically and was changed to oral therapy with plans to continue long-term treatment due to continued immunosuppressive therapy. The finding of *Aspergillus flavus* was important not only to establish a diagnosis of invasive pulmonary aspergillosis but also because of the fact that this species can demonstrate reduced susceptibility to the polyenes.

Recent Developments

Recent outcomes of invasive pulmonary aspergillosis have been improved compared to historical rates even in severely immunosuppressed patients. The reasons for this improvement are unknown but are likely related to antifungal agents like voriconazole that are highly active against *Aspergillus*; improved and aggressive attempts at establishing a diagnosis; early recognition of infection; as well as improved supportive care and immunosuppressive regimens. The use of initial combination therapy was not utilized in this patient. Current recommendations suggest that combination therapy be reserved at the present time for salvage therapy or those not responding to initial therapy. A clinical trial evaluating voriconazole plus an echinocandin (anidulafungin) is completing enrollment and should provide useful data for management guidelines.

Conclusion

This highly immunosuppressed patient was at significant risk for invasive fungal infection. Management should include:

1   Assessment of risk for invasive pulmonary Aspergillus or other fungal pathogen.
2   Aggressive attempts at diagnosis through non-culture-based assays, radiology and BAL to establish a mycological diagnosis.
3   Empirical use of voriconazole as primary therapy for invasive aspergillosis in most patients.

Therapy should be continued through a good therapeutic response and until immunosuppression resolves or is significantly reduced.

Further Reading

Cornely OA, Maertens J, Bresnik M *et al*. Liposomal amphotericin B as initial therapy for invasive mold infection: a randomized trial comparing a high-loading dose regimen with standard dosing (AmBiLoad trial). *Clin Infect Dis* 2007; **44**: 1289–97.

Maertens J, Theunissen K, Verhoef G *et al*. Galactomannan and computed tomography-based preemptive antifungal therapy in neutropenic patients at high risk for invasive fungal infection: a prospective feasibility study. *Clin Infect Dis* 2005; **41**: 1242–50.

Marr KA, Boeckh M, Carter RA, Kim HW, Corey L. Combination antifungal therapy for invasive aspergillosis. *Clin Infect Dis* 2004; **39**: 797–802.

Patterson TF, Boucher HW, Herbrecht R *et al.* Strategy of following voriconazole versus amphotericin B therapy with other licensed antifungal therapy for primary treatment of invasive aspergillosis: impact of other therapies on outcome. *Clin Infect Dis* 2005; **41**: 1448–52.

Patterson TF, Kirkpatrick WR, White M *et al.* Invasive aspergillosis. Disease spectrum, treatment practices, and outcomes. I3 Aspergillus Study Group. *Medicine (Baltimore)* 2000; **79**: 250–60.

Walsh TJ, Anaissie EJ, Denning DW *et al.* Treatment of aspergillosis: clinical practice guidelines of the Infectious Diseases Society of America. *Clin Infect Dis* 2008; **46**: 327–60.

PROBLEM

40 Management of Febrile Neutropenia

Kevin Kerr

Case History

A 42-year-old man was receiving mitoxantrone and cytarabine consolidation chemotherapy as part of treatment for acute myeloid leukaemia. He had been admitted to the ward with rigors and a temperature of 38.7°C, which followed flushing of his Hickman line. He had no cough or sore throat and no symptoms of urinary frequency or dysuria. There had been no diarrhoea and he denied perianal tenderness. He was not known to be a carrier of methicillin-resistant *Staphylococcus aureus* (MRSA). Physical examination was unremarkable; the Hickman line exit site, in particular, showed no erythema or exudate. A full blood count revealed a neutrophil count of $0.2 \times 10^9/l$. Blood cultures were obtained from each lumen of the line and a peripheral vein, as well as a swab from the Hickman line exit site. A mid-stream specimen of urine was taken, after which he was commenced on piperacillin-tazobactam and gentamicin. The following day he remained pyrexial. On the third day of admission the microbiology laboratory reported that the blood cultures obtained from the Hickman line contained a Gram-negative bacillus (Figure 40.1). Later that day, Gram-negative bacilli were also noted in the peripheral blood cultures. Cultures from the line exit site were reported as 'skin flora only'.

How should this patient now be managed in the context of the microbiology results?

Why did the patient develop the infection?

How might this infection have been prevented?

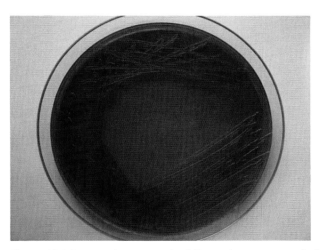

Figure 40.1 *Stenotrophomonas maltophilia* growing on vancomycin-imipenem-amphotericin B (VIA) agar. Other imipenem-resistant Gram-negative bacteria produce acid from mannitol contained in the agar, resulting in yellow colonies; this is not demonstrated by *S. maltophilia* where no colour change is observed (courtesy of Ms Claire Wright, University of Bradford) (*see inside front cover for colour version*).

Background

Febrile neutropenia can be defined as fever (a single oral temperature of ≥38.3°C or a temperature ≥38°C sustained over an hour) in a patient with an absolute neutrophil count of <0.5 × 10⁹/l. Febrile neutropenia is a medical emergency and patients should be assessed rapidly and immediately commenced on antimicrobial therapy without waiting for results from microbiological investigations. This is because patients may deteriorate rapidly, with the onset of severe sepsis, and also because cultures are frequently negative. There is a tendency to submit a 'full septic screen' in patients with febrile neutropenia, but specimen submission should be guided by clinical signs and symptoms. All patients with febrile neutropenia should have at least two sets of blood cultures taken from a peripheral vein and from each lumen of any venous access device present. If cultures subsequently become positive, differential times to positivity can be measured. A highly sensitive and specific indicator for catheter-related bacteraemia occurs when catheter cultures become positive more than two hours before peripheral specimens (i.e. differential time to positivity >2 hours).

There is a need for broad-spectrum empirical therapy given that a wide range of microorganisms may cause fever in a neutropenic patient; this is compounded by the fact that clinical signs and symptoms are often insufficient to identify a focus of infection.

Every centre managing patients that receive potentially myelosuppressive therapy should have policies and protocols for empirical and ongoing antimicrobial therapy of febrile neutropenia. The agents recommended in these policies should take into account local epidemiology and resistance patterns and will thus vary from centre to centre. Irrespective of these differences the general principles of empirical therapy are to employ a broad-spectrum agent that includes activity against *Pseudomonas aeruginosa*, e.g. carbapenems such as imipenem or meropenem, and anti-pseudomonal β-lactams, including cefepime, ceftazidime or piperacillin-tazobactam. In some centres a second agent, usually an aminoglycoside such as gentamicin, is added, although a meta-analysis has shown that monotherapy is equivalent to combination regimens regarding efficacy. Initial treatment may require modification depending on clinical features or if the patient has a history of colonization or infection with multiresistant bacteria that would not otherwise be 'covered' by first-line therapy. For example, metronidazole would be added to ceftazidime if the patient had signs and symptoms suggestive of perianal infection caused by anaerobic bacteria. Similarly, standard empirical therapy would be supplemented with a glycopeptide, e.g. vancomycin or teicoplanin, if the patient was known to be colonized with MRSA.

Management

The patient was commenced on piperacillin-tazobactam and gentamicin on admission but remained pyrexial the following day. This might have indicated that the causative bacterium was resistant to these agents, but the fact that the blood culture isolates flagged positive before peripherally obtained specimens suggested a Hickman line-associated infection. Many types of bacteria can cause these infections ranging from Gram-positive bacteria, including staphylococci and *Corynebacterium* spp. (colloquially referred to as 'diphtheroids'), Gram-negative bacteria and yeasts such as *Candida*. The ability to form biofilm is a characteristic of many microorganisms which cause line infections. Biofilm refers to an aggregate of cells embedded in an extracellular matrix and is often referred to as 'slime'. Biofilm-associated bacteria adhere to the extra- and intraluminal surfaces of the line and are difficult to eradicate using conventional antimicrobial therapy.

If the infection is caused by pathogens of limited virulence, for example coagulase-negative staphylococci (usually *Staphylococcus epidermidis*) or *Corynebacterium* spp., attempts can be made to salvage the line using intraluminal antibiotic or 'lock' therapy. Here, a solution of an antibiotic at very high concentration is introduced into the catheter lumen and allowed to dwell for several hours; the rationale is that sufficient antimicrobial will passively diffuse through the biofilm to achieve concentrations that will kill adherent bacteria. If organisms of greater pathogenicity – e.g. Gram-negative bacteria, *S. aureus* and fungi – are identified as the cause of line infection, then lock therapy is better avoided. Under these circumstances successful management of the infection relies on removal of the line in conjunction with appropriate antimicrobial therapy. In this case, since the differential time to positivity suggested a line-associated infection caused by Gram-negative bacteria, the consultant microbiologist recommended that the line should be removed, particularly as the patient was still spiking high fevers with rigors.

Outcome

The line was removed and the patient's condition improved significantly. The blood culture bacterium (and also from the tip of the removed Hickman line) was identified as *Stenotrophomonas maltophilia*. As this isolate was resistant to both piperacillin-tazobactam and gentamicin, the patient's response was almost certainly due to removal of the line, thus highlighting the importance of line manipulation in cases of line-associated infection caused by Gram-negative bacteria. *S. maltophilia* (previously *Pseudomonas* or *Xanthomonas maltophilia*) is an environmental bacterium which is increasingly recognized as a cause of infection in immunocompromised individuals. Management of infections caused by *S. maltophilia* is problematic because the bacterium manifests inherent or acquired resistance to many broad-spectrum antimicrobials. It is always resistant to carbapenems. Moreover, there are a number of pitfalls in relation to *in vivo* susceptibility testing, as results are affected both by temperature of incubation and the testing medium used and there is no good correlation between *in vitro* susceptibility and clinical outcome. Co-trimoxazole (trimethoprim plus sulfamethoxazole) is the drug of choice for *S. maltophilia* infection, although this is less than ideal in neutropenic patients given the potential myelosuppressive properties of this combination.

Recent Developments

Prevention of infection

The practice of giving antimicrobial prophylaxis, usually with a fluoroquinolone such as ciprofloxacin, for patients who become neutropenic varies from centre to centre and has been the subject of much debate. Critics of this approach are concerned about the use of a therapeutically important class of drugs in this way and cite the risk of superinfection with microorganisms that are quinolone resistant.

Other infection-prevention strategies include 'reverse barrier nursing' during periods of neutropenia and, to reduce exposure to environmental Gram-negative bacteria including *S. maltophilia* and *P. aeruginosa*, removal of plants and fresh flowers from patient care areas as well as avoidance of certain foodstuffs, e.g. pre-packaged salads. To minimize the risk of line-associated infection, central venous lines should be inserted by experienced operators using maximal barrier precautions and, once *in situ*, lines should be accessed under strict aseptic conditions.

Conclusion

Infection remains a major cause of morbidity and mortality in patients rendered neutropenic following treatment for both solid organ and haematological malignancy. Successful management depends on timely assessment of patients after they present and prompt institution of broad-spectrum antimicrobials. Neutropenic patients are prone to infection with a very wide range of microorganisms including environmental, 'opportunist' bacteria which are uncommonly associated with sepsis in non-immunosuppressed individuals. Many environmental bacteria are multiply antibiotic resistant, which complicates the management of the infections that they cause. Line-associated infection in neutropenic infections responds poorly to antimicrobial therapy and a successful outcome is usually achieved only by removing the line.

Further Reading

de Naurois NJ, Novitzky-Basso I, Gill MJ, Marti FM, Cullen MH, Roila F. Management of febrile neutropenia: ESMO Clinical Practice Guidelines. *Ann Oncol* 2010; **21**(Suppl 5): v252–6.

Denton M, Kerr KG. Microbiological and clinical aspects of infection associated with *Stenotrophomonas maltophilia*. *Clin Microbiol Rev* 1998; **11**: 57–80.

Freifeld AG, Bow EJ, Sepkowitz KA *et al*. Clinical practice guideline for the use of antimicrobial agents in neutropenic patients with cancer: 2010 update by the Infectious Diseases Society of America. *Clin Infect Dis* 2011; **52**: e56–93.

Pascoe J, Steven N. Antibiotics for the prevention of febrile neutropenia. *Curr Opin Hematol* 2009; **16**: 48–52.

Raad I, Hanna H, Maki D. Intravascular catheter-related infections: advances in diagnosis, prevention, and management. *Lancet Infect Dis* 2007; **7**: 645–57.

PROBLEM

41 Catheter-related Bloodstream Infection

Stephen Barrett

Case History

A 70-year-old man had a colonic resection for carcinoma of the sigmoid colon with fashioning of an ileostomy. After four months, a two-lumen Hickman line was inserted for chemotherapy. Three weeks into his chemotherapy he developed a chest infection which was treated with co-amoxiclav. One week later he complained of feeling generally unwell and had low-grade pyrexia. His white blood cell count was $4.8 \times 10^9/l$ and C-reactive protein (CRP) was 28 mg/l. A blood culture taken through the Hickman line yielded coagulase-negative staphylococci (CNS) in one of the two bottles; the organism was resistant to clindamycin, erythromycin and methicillin, and sensitive to fusidic acid, teicoplanin and vancomycin.

How can you establish the significance of this result?

What might be the source of the staphylococci?

If it is significant, how could the infection be treated?

Background

CNS are the commonest organisms isolated from blood cultures. This reflects their ubiquitous nature as skin flora and their ability to persist in the environment when shed on skin squames, etc. They are thus the most likely bacteria to contaminate imperfectly collected blood cultures. They are therefore generally dismissed as insignificant and, in contrast to most other isolates from blood cultures, a case has to be made that they are significant in an individual patient, rather than that they are not.

CNS do not have the same ability to produce exotoxins and other virulence factors that characterize infections by *Staphylococcus aureus* and are rarely pathogenic. Generally the only circumstances in which they may be significant in blood cultures is in the presence of implanted devices, such as intravascular lines, joint prostheses, artificial cardiac valves, etc. Here, their ability to colonize surfaces and grow in impenetrable biofilms, coupled with their frequent antibiotic multiresistance and widespread presence on the skin and as airborne contaminants, gives them the opportunity to establish infection. Patients do not experience severe sepsis due to CNS, but more usually indolent infections with low-grade pyrexia and, in prolonged cases, immune complex disease along with eventual failure of the infected device.

In the case of Mr H described above, the only recognizable focus for a CNS infection is his Hickman line. His feeling unwell could be due to his underlying disease and treatment, or to a low-grade CNS infection of his line. The lack of a raised white blood cell count could be due to his chemotherapy, but the white cell count does not always rise greatly with CNS infections. The pyrexia suggests an infection may be present, although the possibility of its being due to his underlying disease or treatment needs considering, and the slightly raised CRP is problematic to interpret. The overall clinical picture is therefore ambiguous. Isolating the CNS in only one of the two blood culture bottles adds to the uncertainty. Blood cultures cannot normally be quantified, and a positive result may be due to a heavy bacteraemia, or simply a single organism introduced extraneously. If both bottles were positive, this would at least suggest more than a single contaminating bacterial cell, but in itself would not disprove contamination.

Further investigation

The sample for the two blood culture bottles had been collected through a single lumen of the Hickman line. Inspection of the line exit site showed no evidence of infection. The possibilities therefore are that there is colonization of the connector hub of that lumen, or that there may be genuine infection of the line, or that the positive blood culture was merely contaminated. To establish which of these is the case will clearly require the taking of more blood cultures. A genuine infection of the line would be expected to involve the intravascular tip and to affect both lumina, and so blood cultures taken through each of them should yield the same result. In addition, one would expect the infection to result in a bacteraemia causing the same organism to be found in blood cultures collected via a peripheral venepuncture.

Because of the patient's clinical condition, further sets of blood cultures, each of two blood culture bottles, were collected through each connector hub and from an antecubital venepuncture. After 24 hours both bottles collected through the lumen which originally yielded a positive result gave a growth of CNS with the same antibiotic sensitivities as previously. The pattern of antibiotic sensitivities (antibiogram) displayed by CNS can be important circumstantial evidence as to whether one is dealing with the same or a different strain. Patients are often colonized by multiple strains and these may have a variety of antibiograms.

One bottle from the peripheral venepuncture yielded a CNS which differed from the original only in that it was resistant to fusidic acid. The other bottles were all negative. The repeat finding of the same CNS suggests there is a true problem with the original lumen since the CNS has been recovered from it on more than one occasion. However, the negative culture from the other lumen suggests that this problem may be limited to the hub connector. The single positive bottle from the distant venepuncture site leaves the question of line infection unresolved. Although a CNS has been isolated, its susceptibility is not identical with the first isolate. However, it differs in a single antibiotic susceptibility of those tested, and CNS not infrequently contain subpopulations that give minor differences in antibiotic susceptibility patterns. It might therefore represent the same organism, but its finding in only a single bottle suggests a minimal bacteraemia or even contamination. If the patient indeed has a connector hub colonization with this

CNS, then it is probably to be found amongst his skin flora and so could easily have contaminated the peripheral venepuncture anyway.

Management

The patient began to experience sudden episodes of hypotension, collapse and pyrexia. Although it was unclear whether this was due to line infection or sepsis elsewhere, the patient was placed on vancomycin and broad-spectrum antibiotics; the line was removed and his temperature spikes resolved (Figure 41.1). The removed line was cut into segments and cultured on agar using the 'roll' technique. This showed a gradient of increasing CNS colonization from the tip towards the exit site (Figure 41.2).

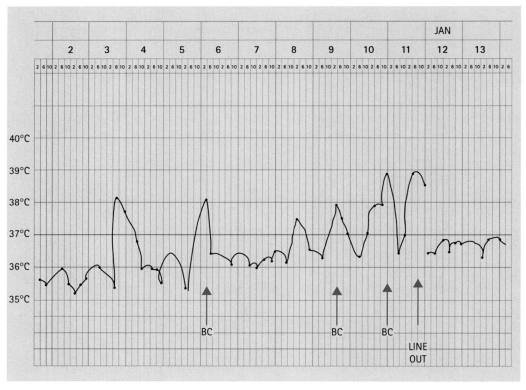

Figure 41.1 Temperature chart showing sudden resolution of pyrexia upon removal of the Hickman line. BC, time blood culture taken.

Removal of an infected line is undoubtedly the most effective form of treatment, but may be a difficult decision if it requires replacement in a debilitated patient. For this reason attempts are sometimes made to preserve the line using antibiotics, particularly if it is only required for a short time longer. 'Antibiotic lock' is a common approach to this with CNS infections. Vancomycin or teicoplanin is infused into the lumen of the line and is left there when the line is not in use. In some cases this appears to eliminate the infection, and generally at least suppresses the CNS. For more virulent bacteria such as

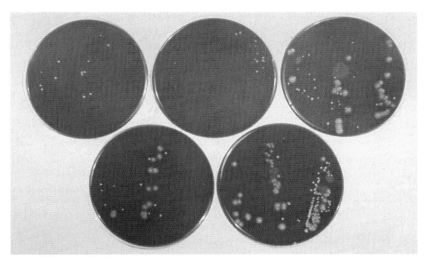

Figure 41.2 'Roll' plate of removed Hickman line. Fifteen equally spaced segments of the line were rolled on blood agar plates and an increasing gradient of contamination can be seen from the intravascular tip (top left) to the exit site (bottom right).

Staphylococcus aureus and Gram-negative bacilli, or for *Candida* sp., systemic antibiotics, even after removal of the line, may be recommended.

Further Considerations

 Other diagnostic approaches have been tried. Quantitative methods, in which the numbers of bacteria isolated through the line are compared with those from a peripheral culture, have been found to predict infection, as has the rate of growth in cultures taken from the two sites. At a preventive level, antimicrobial-impregnated lines have been found to be of some benefit.

Conclusion

 This case illustrates the practical difficulties frequently encountered in deciding whether a line is infected. The laboratory could not provide the sophisticated techniques that might have resolved the uncertainty, and the patient was not severely ill. Since the line was not required for much longer, the pragmatic approach was to remove it. Had it been more important to continue with the line, suppressive treatment with an antibiotic lock might have been attempted.

Further Reading

 O'Grady NP, Alexander M, Dellinger EP *et al.* Guidelines for the prevention of intravascular catheter-related infections. Centers for Disease Control and Prevention. *MMWR Recomm Rep* 2002; **51**(RR-10): 1–29.

Pratt RJ, Pellowe CM, Wilson JA *et al.* epic2: National evidence-based guidelines for preventing healthcare-associated infections in NHS hospitals in England. *J Hosp Infect* 2007; **65**(Suppl 1): S1–64.

Raad I, Hanna H, Maki D. Intravascular catheter-related infections: advances in diagnosis, prevention, and management. *Lancet Infect Dis* 2007; **7**: 645–57.

THE RETURNING TRAVELLER

PROBLEM

42 Severe Malaria

Claire Mackintosh

Case History

A 22-year-old woman presented to the accident and emergency department with a 24-hour history of fever, rigors and headache. She had returned from a three-month backpacking trip in East Africa one week before. She reported receiving all advised pre-travel vaccinations and took doxycycline as malaria prophylaxis. On closer questioning she admitted stopping the doxycycline when she arrived at the Kenyan coast ten days prior to returning to the UK due to photosensitivity concerns. On examination she was alert, tanned, mildly jaundiced and had multiple healing mosquito bites over both calves. She was febrile at 38.8°C and her respiratory rate was 28 breaths/min with an oxygen saturation on air of 90%. Her heart rate was 110 bpm and her blood pressure was 100/60 mmHg. Examination of her chest revealed bibasal inspiratory crackles. Investigations revealed a platelet count of 60/ml³, haemoglobin of 7.8 g/dl, bilirubin of 90 μmol/l and creatinine of 169 μmol/l. Arterial blood gas sampling revealed a lactate of 3.5 mmol/l with a hydrogen ion of 60 nmol/l. The rapid diagnostic test (RDT) for malaria antigen was positive and a subsequent Giemsa-stained blood film revealed the presence of numerous ring forms of *Plasmodium falciparum* with a parasitaemia of 2%.

In what clinical area should this patient be managed?

What should her initial therapy consist of?

If her haemodynamic parameters do not improve following fluid resuscitation, what additional diagnoses should be considered?

Background

Malaria is a risk to around 2.1 billion individuals in over 100 countries. An estimated 30 000 international travellers fall ill with the disease annually. In the UK, between 1500 and 2000 cases are reported each year, three-quarters of which are due to *Plasmodium falciparum*. Over two-thirds of cases occur in people of African or Asian origin returning from visiting friends and family in endemic areas, with West Africa the most common area of acquisition of *P. falciparum*.

Patients presenting with *P. falciparum* can exhibit a range of clinical features from mild non-specific symptoms such as headache, malaise and general lethargy to severe life-threatening illness. Fever does not invariably exist at time of presentation. Clinical suspicion is paramount and the diagnosis should be considered in any returning traveller. The minimum incubation period for *P. falciparum* is six days and patients can present up to six months following exposure.

Severe malaria, predominantly caused by *P. falciparum*, is a complex multisystem disorder presenting with a range of clinical features. The development of severe malaria is as a result of a combination of parasite-specific factors – adhesion and sequestration in the vasculature and the release of bioactive molecules – together with host inflammatory responses. Patient groups most at risk for developing severe disease include children, pregnant women and the elderly.

Management

All patients with *P. falciparum* malaria should be admitted to hospital. In those in whom the diagnosis is suspected but where initial RDT or blood films are negative, the investigations should be repeated twice within the subsequent 48 hours. Empirical treatment for malaria should not be commenced unless a relevant exposure history is accompanied

---

Box 42.1 Assessing the signs of severe malaria.

Features of severe malaria in adults
- Renal impairment
- Impaired consciousness/seizures
- Acidosis (pH <7.3)
- Hypoglycaemia
- Anaemia (haemoglobin <8 g/dl)
- Coagulopathy
- Pulmonary oedema/adult respiratory distress syndrome
- Haemodynamic compromise (systolic blood pressure <90 mmHg, heart rate >100 beats/min)

Other situations of concern
- Pregnant women
- Hyperparasitaemia (≥2%)
- Elderly patients (>65 years)
- Persistent vomiting

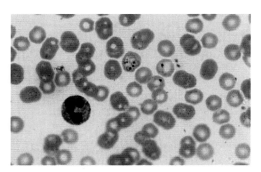

Figure 42.1 Photomicrograph of a peripheral blood film showing the presence of *P. falciparum* including evidence of red blood cells infected with multiple ring forms.

with signs of severe disease and expert advice has been taken. Patients presenting with *P. falciparum* malaria should be assessed for signs of severe disease (Box 42.1). These include impaired conscious level, renal impairment, pulmonary oedema or respiratory distress, anaemia, impaired clotting time, features of haemodynamic collapse, hypoglycaemia and acidosis. Other laboratory markers of severe illness include a peripheral parasitaemia of greater than 2%, the presence of peripherally circulating schizonts on a blood film (Figure 42.1) and an elevated lactate. If any of these markers are present, the patient should be managed in a critical care or high-dependency setting.

In those individuals with no signs of severe or complicated disease, initial therapy should consist of one of the following options: oral artesunate 2 mg/kg daily plus doxycycline (or clindamycin in pregnant patients) or atovaquone-proguanil (Malarone®) or artemether-lumefantrin (Coartem®/Riamet®). The first option must be given for five to seven days with the second agent given either concurrently or sequentially. This is required in order to ensure parasite clearance. The second option is given for a total of three days and no second agent is required.

If features of severe disease are present, or the patient is at high risk of developing severe disease (pregnant women, peripheral parasitaemia greater than 2%), or in those unable to tolerate oral medication, there should be no delay in administering urgent, appropriate parenteral therapy. The first-line therapy in the UK remains intravenous artesunate. IV artesunate is given in four equal doses of 2.4 mg/kg over a period of three days. The dosing schedule recommended by the World Health Organization (WHO) entails doses every 12 hours on day 1 and then once daily. Therapy for more than three days may occasionally be indicated in very ill patients. Artesunate dosages need not be changed because of hepatic or renal failure or concomitant or previous therapy with other medications, including previous therapy with mefloquine, quinine, or quinidine. There are no known interactions between artesunate and other drugs.

Following initial IV treatment, once the patient can tolerate oral therapy, it is essential to continue and complete treatment with an effective oral antimalarial drug combination such as: artesunate plus amodiaquine; or artemether plus lumefantrine; or dihydroartemisinin plus piperaquine; or artesunate plus clindamycin or doxycycline. Clindamycin may be substituted in children and pregnant women as doxycycline cannot be given to these groups.

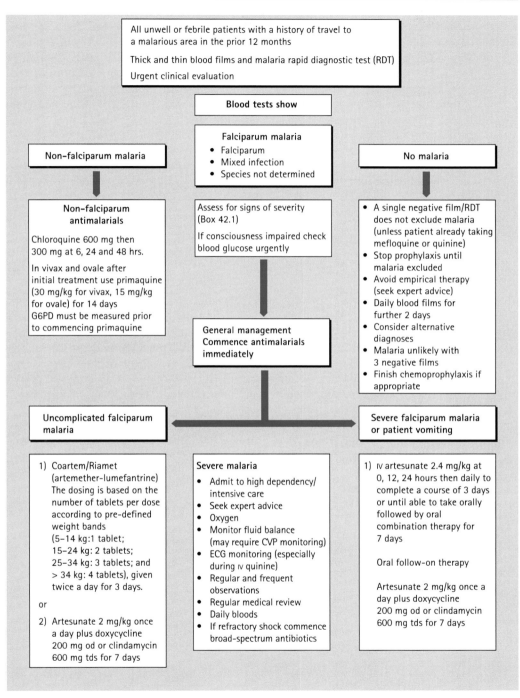

All unwell or febrile patients with a history of travel to a malarious area in the prior 12 months

Thick and thin blood films and malaria rapid diagnostic test (RDT)

Urgent clinical evaluation

Blood tests show

Falciparum malaria
- Falciparum
- Mixed infection
- Species not determined

Non–falciparum malaria

No malaria

Non–falciparum antimalarials

Chloroquine 600 mg then 300 mg at 6, 24 and 48 hrs.

In vivax and ovale after initial treatment use primaquine (30 mg/kg for vivax, 15 mg/kg for ovale) for 14 days
G6PD must be measured prior to commencing primaquine

Assess for signs of severity (Box 42.1)

If consciousness impaired check blood glucose urgently

- A single negative film/RDT does not exclude malaria (unless patient already taking mefloquine or quinine)
- Stop prophylaxis until malaria excluded
- Avoid empirical therapy (seek expert advice)
- Daily blood films for further 2 days
- Consider alternative diagnoses
- Malaria unlikely with 3 negative films
- Finish chemoprophylaxis if appropriate

**General management
Commence antimalarials immediately**

Uncomplicated falciparum malaria

Severe falciparum malaria or patient vomiting

1) Coartem/Riamet (artemether–lumefantrine) The dosing is based on the number of tablets per dose according to pre-defined weight bands (5–14 kg:1 tablet; 15–24 kg: 2 tablets; 25–34 kg: 3 tablets; and > 34 kg: 4 tablets), given twice a day for 3 days.

or

2) Artesunate 2 mg/kg once a day plus doxycycline 200 mg od or clindamycin 600 mg tds for 7 days

Severe malaria
- Admit to high dependency/intensive care
- Seek expert advice
- Oxygen
- Monitor fluid balance (may require CVP monitoring)
- ECG monitoring (especially during IV quinine)
- Regular and frequent observations
- Regular medical review
- Daily bloods
- If refractory shock commence broad-spectrum antibiotics

1) IV artesunate 2.4 mg/kg at 0, 12, 24 hours then daily to complete a course of 3 days or until able to take orally followed by oral combination therapy for 7 days

Oral follow-on therapy

Artesunate 2 mg/kg once a day plus doxycycline 200 mg od or clindamycin 600 mg tds for 7 days

Figure 42.2 An algorithm for the management of suspected malaria (adapted from British Infection Society guidelines, 2007). CVP, central venous pressure; ECG, electrocardiogram; G6PD, glucose 6-phosphate dehydrogenase.

Additional supportive measures should be instituted as appropriate. Accurate fluid balance should be maintained with the aid of central venous monitoring as required. Hypoglycaemia can occur as a consequence of severe malaria or as a result of quinine-induced hyperinsulinaemia and regular blood glucose monitoring should be performed.

Frequent parasite counts are not helpful in the early management of severe malaria with the peripheral parasite count fluctuating according to the stage of parasite development. It is thus not uncommon for the parasite count to increase in the first 24 hours of treatment. Daily parasite counts are therefore sufficient.

If patients have signs of shock and these do not improve with initial fluid balance correction, a broad-spectrum antibiotic should be commenced. In one recent study, 62% of bacteraemia cases were attributable to co-infection with malaria. In one study, concurrent bacteraemia was identified in 7%–14% of patients admitted with severe malaria. There is no evidence for the use of steroids in the management of severe malaria, and the use of exchange transfusion is controversial and should only be undertaken after discussion with an expert (Figure 42.2).

Recent Developments

With the ultimate aim of reducing and eventually eliminating the considerable global burden of disease inflicted by malaria, there are a number of promising vaccine candidates showing evidence of benefit in field studies. Trials of the RTS, S vaccine have shown 46% protection persisting over 15 months of follow-up amongst Kenyan infants. Recent preliminary data from a vaccine safety study using the blood-stage antigen MSP3, have demonstrated a substantial reduction in malaria incidence, albeit in a small number of individuals.

Thanks to a huge increase in international funding for malaria control, the last 10 years has seen a large reduction in both malaria cases and deaths. The WHO World Malaria Report of 2010 found that in eleven countries this reduction has been in excess of 50%. The challenge for the future is in maintaining and improving on these impressive gains. History has shown that when malaria-endemic countries scale back their control activities, malaria quickly resurges.

Further Reading

Artemeter-Quinine Meta-analysis Study Group. A meta-analysis using individual patient data of trials comparing artemether with quinine in the treatment of severe falciparum malaria. *Trans R Soc Trop Med Hyg* 2001; **95**: 637–50.

Bejon PB, Lusingu J, Olotu A *et al.* Efficacy of RTS,S/AS01E vaccine against malaria in children 5 to 17 months of age. *N Engl J Med* 2008; **359**: 2521–32.

Berkley J, Mwarumba S, Bramham K, Lowe B, Marsh K. Bacteraemia complicating severe malaria in children. *Trans R Soc Trop Med Hyg* 1999; **93**: 283–6.

Day NP, Phu NH, Mai NT *et al.* The pathophysiologic and prognostic significance of acidosis in severe adult malaria. *Crit Care Med* 2000; **28**: 1833–40.

Dondorp A, Nosten F, Stepniewska K, Day N, White N; South East Asian Quinine Artesunate Malaria Trial (SEAQUAMAT) group. Artesunate versus quinine for treatment of severe falciparum malaria: a randomised trial. *Lancet* 2005; **366**: 717–25.

Jones KL, Donegan S, Lalloo DG. Artesunate versus quinine for treating severe malaria. *Cochrane Database Syst Rev* 2007; CD005967.

Lalloo DG, Shingadia D, Pasvol G *et al*. UK malaria treatment guidelines. *J Infect* 2007; **54**: 111–21.

Mackintosh CL, Beeson JG, Marsh K. Clinical features and pathogenesis of severe malaria. *Trends Parasitol* 2004; **20**: 597–603.

Riddle MS, Jackson JL, Sanders JW, Blazes DL. Exchange transfusion as an adjunct therapy in severe Plasmodium falciparum malaria: a meta-analysis. *Clin Infect Dis* 2002; **34**: 1192–8.

Scott JAG, Berkley JA, Mwangi I *et al*. Relation between falciparum malaria and bacteraemia in Kenyan children: a population-based, case control study and a longitudinal study. *Lancet* 2011; **378**: 1316–23.

Sirima SB, Cousens S, Druilhe P. Protection against malaria by MSP3 candidate vaccine. *N Engl J Med* 2011; **365**: 1062–4.

Snow RW, Guerra CA, Noor AM, Myint HY, Hay SI. The global distribution of clinical episodes of Plasmodium falciparum malaria. *Nature* 2005; **434**: 214–17.

Warrell DA, Looareesuwan S, Warrell MJ *et al*. Dexamethasone proves deleterious in cerebral malaria. A double-blind trial in 100 comatose patients. *N Engl J Med* 1982; **306**: 313–19.

World Health Organization. World Malaria Report 2010. Available at: http://www.who.int/malaria/world_malaria_report_2010/en/index.html (accessed 13 10 11).

PROBLEM

43 Melioidosis

Bart J. Currie

Case History

A 29-year-old male returned to the UK from a backpacking holiday in Northern Australia. During the flight home he developed fevers and abdominal pain and he noted some dysuria and mild diarrhoea. On presentation to the emergency department the next day he felt worse, his temperature was 39.5°C and on examination he had a non-specifically tender abdomen and appeared to be in urinary retention. A urinary catheter was inserted, draining 750 ml of slightly dark urine, blood cultures were taken as well as standard blood tests and he was commenced on intravenous ampicillin, gentamicin and metronidazole.

The next day he remained febrile and unwell. The microbiology laboratory reported growth of a Gram-negative bacillus from both his blood cultures and urine.

What is the likely diagnosis?

What further investigations should be done?

What do you recommend as therapy?

Background

This is a classical presentation of melioidosis with genitourinary infection and prostatic abscess(es). The case illustrates the importance of a good travel and activity history in returned travellers who present with a febrile illness.

Melioidosis is caused by infection with the soil and water bacterium *Burkholderia pseudomallei*. It is thought to usually follow percutaneous inoculation, but inhalation of aerosolized bacteria may occur during tropical storms. Melioidosis following aspiration is also documented, such as occurred with the 2004 Asian tsunami and also following vehicular accidents with near drowning. Zoonotic transmission is exceedingly uncommon, as are person-to-person transmission and laboratory-acquired infection. Mortality from melioidosis remains over 50% in some endemic locations, but is under 20% in situations where early diagnosis occurs, appropriate antibiotics are administered and high-level intensive care management is available for patients with severe sepsis.

Most cases of melioidosis in returned travellers have been acquired in the traditional melioidosis-endemic regions of Southeast Asia and Northern Australia. However, the boundaries of endemicity for environmental presence of *B. pseudomallei* remain unclear, with recent case reports of melioidosis from Madagascar, Mauritius, India, China, Taiwan, and South and Central American countries including Brazil and the Caribbean.

Activities that should be asked about in returned travellers that suggest possible infecting events include exposure to muddy soils and water in melioidosis-endemic locations, especially during the monsoonal wet season. Adventure holidays with camping or walking in such environments have preceded melioidosis cases presenting in Europe, the United States and Southern Australia. In addition, occupational exposure in endemic locations has resulted in melioidosis in returning expatriate mine workers and others with similar outdoor jobs. Melioidosis also needs to be considered in residents of melioidosis-endemic regions who become unwell after travelling to non-endemic countries.

Serological surveys indicate that the majority of infections with *B. pseudomallei* are asymptomatic, with over half of teenagers seropositive in northeast Thailand. It is evident that certain risk factors strongly predispose the infected person to developing clinical disease (i.e. melioidosis). Most notable is diabetes (both types 1 and 2 diabetes), with up to 60% of cases in some series being diabetic. Other important risk factors for melioidosis are chronic lung disease, excessive alcohol intake, renal disease, thalassaemia, malignancy and immunosuppressive therapy. An increasing number of recent reports of melioidosis in people with cystic fibrosis travelling to Southeast Asia and Northern Australia has prompted calls for those with cystic fibrosis to avoid travel to locations where melioidosis is common. Nevertheless, 20%–36% of patients with melioidosis have no identified predisposing risk factor.

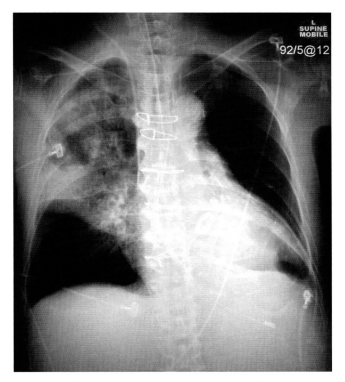

Figure 43.1 Chest X-ray showing fatal septicaemic melioidosis pneumonia.

Melioidosis has a large diversity of presentations and any organ system can be involved. The spectrum of illness ranges from innocuous skin ulcers or crusted lesions to septicaemia with multiple internal organ abscesses with high mortality. Around 40%–60% of patients are blood culture-positive for *B. pseudomallei*. Overall, half of all cases present with pneumonia, which can be part of a fatal septicaemia, a less severe unilateral infection indistinguishable from other community-acquired pneumonias or a chronic illness mimicking tuberculosis (Figure 43.1). Genitourinary, bone, joint and neurological presentations are also well recognized. Three differences between case series from Thailand and Northern Australia are the higher frequency of parotid abscesses in Thai children with melioidosis and the higher rates of prostatic and neurological melioidosis in Australia. Primary neurological melioidosis in Australia is manifested usually by a meningo-encephalitic syndrome, often with cranial nerve palsies from brainstem involvement. Patients can also present with predominantly spinal cord involvement, with fever, flaccid paraparesis and urinary retention. In addition to the primary clinical presentation, secondary clinical features are also common, usually resulting from bacteraemic spread of *B. pseudomallei*. Hence, secondary pneumonia after another primary presentation can occur in around 10% of cases, and secondary septic arthritis, osteomyelitis and abscesses in prostate and brain all occur. Overall, prostatic abscesses are found in around 20% of Australian males with melioidosis, with most having a primary genitourinary presentation as in the case described here.

Investigation and management

The likelihood of diagnosing melioidosis is maximized if the diagnosis is considered in at-risk subjects and appropriate clinical samples are sent to the microbiology laboratory. A definitive diagnosis of melioidosis is made when *B. pseudomallei* is cultured from a clinical sample such as blood, sputum, urine, wound or abscess swab or pus, or throat or rectal swab inserted into selective culture media such as Ashdown's medium (a gentamicin-containing liquid broth) or *Burkholderia cepacia* medium. Laboratories inexperienced with *B. pseudomallei* may have difficulty identifying the recovered Gram-negative organism, so notifying the laboratory of the suspicion of possible melioidosis is helpful. Serology is only available in selected laboratories, does not provide definitive diagnosis and may be negative early in melioidosis sepsis and positive in many healthy people living in endemic locations. Nevertheless, positive melioidosis serology in a sick returned traveller who has visited but is not usually resident in an endemic area warrants consideration of further assessment.

Once melioidosis is diagnosed, the definitive antibiotic therapy consists of an intensive phase of intravenous ceftazidime or meropenem, usually for a minimum of two weeks, followed by an eradication phase of oral therapy, usually with co-trimoxazole with or without doxycycline, usually for a further three months. The organism is inherently resistant to gentamicin. Co-trimoxazole is added to the intravenous therapy in the intensive phase when infection involves the brain, prostate, bone and joints.

With careful follow-up and adherence to therapy, relapse of melioidosis and development of acquired antimicrobial resistance are very uncommon, with cure and eradication of infection expected. Secondary undiagnosed foci of infection such as internal abscesses and bone and joint melioidosis may be responsible for persisting fevers and recrudescence. Due to the propensity for deep infections, a computed tomography scan of the abdomen and pelvis is recommended for all patients where possible to identify internal organ abscesses. In the case described here this would demonstrate prostatic abscess(es) (Figure 43.2). Prostatic abscesses usually require drainage, with initial radiologically guided drainage via a rectal ultrasound being least invasive and often successful. A chest X-ray is required in all patients irrespective of initial clinical presentation.

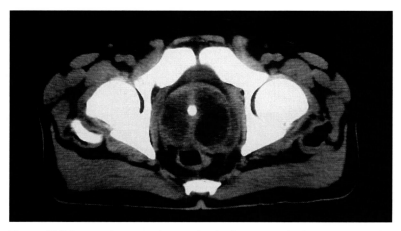

Figure 43.2 Computed tomography scan showing large prostatic abscesses as a result of melioidosis.

Recent Developments

The resurgence of interest in *B. pseudomallei* in the last decade has been largely driven by its recognition as a potential biothreat agent. This has resulted in the genomes of a large number of strains of *B. pseudomallei* being sequenced to assess bacterial diversity and geographical and clinical correlates of specific genomic islands and potential virulence genes of interest. Despite this, and the recognition that melioidosis can be such a dramatically overwhelming infection, specific virulence factors responsible for severe disease remain surprisingly poorly elucidated, as do the specific reasons why diabetes is such an important risk factor for melioidosis.

A number of large, randomized, comparative trials have been undertaken in Thailand to optimize the antibiotic therapy of melioidosis. These have substantially improved outcomes, together with the increased recognition of the infection, enhanced diagnostic capabilities and improved intensive care management of severe sepsis.

Conclusion

Melioidosis should be considered in any febrile traveller returning from or who lives in a melioidosis-endemic region. While infection in Southeast Asia and Northern Australia accounts for the vast majority of cases of melioidosis, a number of other locations are recognized as being endemic for *B. pseudomallei*. The clinical course of melioidosis following infection is likely to be determined by a combination of host risk factors for disease (with diabetes the most important risk factor), mode of infection, infecting dose of bacteria and putative *B. pseudomallei* strain differences in virulence. With prompt diagnosis and appropriate therapy the mortality from melioidosis has substantially decreased in recent years.

Further Reading

Chaowagul W. Recent advances in the treatment of severe melioidosis. *Acta Trop* 2000; **74**: 133–7.

Chaowagul W, Chierakul W, Simpson AJ *et al.* Open-label randomized trial of oral trimethoprim-sulfamethoxazole, doxycycline, and chloramphenicol compared with trimethoprim-sulfamethoxazole and doxycycline for maintenance therapy of melioidosis. *Antimicrob Agents Chemother* 2005; **49**: 4020–5.

Cheng AC, Currie BJ. Melioidosis: epidemiology, pathophysiology, and management. *Clin Microbiol Rev* 2005; **18**: 383–416.

Currie BJ, Fisher DA, Howard DM *et al.* Endemic melioidosis in tropical northern Australia: a 10-year prospective study and review of the literature. *Clin Infect Dis* 2000; **31**: 981–6.

Currie BJ. Melioidosis: an important cause of pneumonia in residents of and travellers returned from endemic regions. *Eur Respir J* 2003; **22**: 542–50.

Currie BJ, Dance DA, Cheng AC. The global distribution of *Burkholderia pseudomallei* and melioidosis: an update. *Trans R Soc Trop Med Hyg* 2008; **102**(Suppl 1): S1–4.

Holden MT, Titball RW, Peacock SJ *et al.* Genomic plasticity of the causative agent of melioidosis, *Burkholderia pseudomallei*. *Proc Natl Acad Sci USA* 2004; **101**: 14240–5.

Inglis TJ, Rolim DB, Sousa Ade Q. Melioidosis in the Americas. *Am J Trop Med Hyg* 2006; **75**: 947–54.

Limmathurotsakul D, Chaowagul W, Chierakul W *et al.* Risk factors for recurrent melioidosis in northeast Thailand. *Clin Infect Dis* 2006; **43**: 979–86.

Morse LP, Moller CC, Harvey E *et al.* Prostatic abscess due to *Burkholderia pseudomallei*: 81 cases from a 19-year prospective melioidosis study. *J Urol* 2009; **182**: 542–7.

Peacock SJ, Schweizer HP, Dance DA *et al.* Management of accidental laboratory exposure to *Burkholderia pseudomallei* and *B. mallei*. *Emerg Infect Dis* 2008; **14**: e2.

White NJ. Melioidosis. *Lancet* 2003; **361**: 1715–22.

Wiersinga WJ, van der Poll T, White NJ, Day NP, Peacock SJ. Melioidosis: insights into the pathogenicity of *Burkholderia pseudomallei*. *Nat Rev Microbiol* 2006; **4**: 272–82.

PROBLEM

44 Acute Febrile Respiratory Illness – Suspected H5N1 Influenza

Lynette Pereira, Dale Fisher

Case History

A 42-year-old man presented to the emergency department with a one-day history of fevers, chills, rigors, myalgias and shortness of breath. He had returned from Vietnam two days earlier, where he had been staying with relatives for a month. One of his relatives had flu-like symptoms just prior to him departing. He was previously fit and healthy with no preceding medical problems. On examination he had a temperature of 38.7°C, a respiratory rate of 28 breaths/min and required 35% oxygen via a mask to maintain his oxygen saturation levels above 90%. Auscultation of his chest revealed widespread bilateral crackles. The chest X-ray performed in the emergency department is shown in Figure 44.1.

What infection control measures should be undertaken at his presentation in the emergency department?

What specimens should be obtained?

How should he be managed?

Background

Emerging pathogenic infections with pandemic potential are a constant source for concern. Current examples include severe acute respiratory syndrome (SARS) and avian

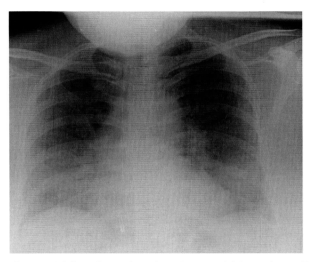

Figure 44.1 Chest X-ray of a patient with acute febrile respiratory illness/ severe acute respiratory syndrome (SARS).

influenza. As shown by SARS in 2003, modern travel facilitates spread causing a threat worldwide (Figure 44.1).

The avian influenza H5N1 virus is highly pathogenic in humans. Most infections in humans have been as a result of close contact with infected poultry with transmission via respiratory routes (predominantly via droplets), but airborne transmission has been proposed. Infection from a contaminated environment and human-to-human transmission has been suspected in patients without apparent direct exposure to poultry. Transmission via the gastrointestinal (GI) tract has also been suspected in patients with initial predominant GI symptoms after consumption of raw poultry.

Human infection with avian influenza usually presents with a typical influenza syndrome with or without GI symptoms, usually two to eight days after exposure. It is thought to be infectious two days before and especially during the first two days of symptoms. Rapid development of complications including acute respiratory distress syndrome (ARDS) and multiorgan failure occurs commonly. Prompt suspicion of avian influenza infection is important for initiating appropriate infection control measures and containing transmission effectively. Although avian influenza is currently not transmitted efficiently from person to person, the possibility of viral mutation changing this, together with its high crude mortality in humans (over 60%), make it a formidable pandemic threat.

Prompt recognition of cases relies on details from the patient's history including recent travel history, occupation and contact with potentially infected persons or poultry. Information on areas where cases of human avian influenza infection have been identified is regularly updated by the World Health Organization (WHO) and is available on their website (http://www.who.int/csr/disease/avian_influenza).

Infection control measures

All employees of healthcare facilities should be aware of universal standard precautions and these should be applied for all patients. For persons with respiratory infections, infection control measures should be implemented from the first point of presentation. The Centers for Disease Control and Prevention (CDC) have published guidelines for the prevention of all respiratory tract infections in healthcare settings and these are available in detail on their website (http://www.cdc.gov/flu).

These guidelines recommend:

- Posting visual alerts in waiting areas where patients first register
- Respiratory hygiene and cough etiquette measures
- Performing hand hygiene after contact with respiratory secretions
- Masking and separation of persons with respiratory symptoms
- Observing droplet precautions

For persons suspected of infection with highly pathogenic novel organisms or avian influenza because of clinical symptoms and epidemiological risk factors, such as the case for the patient described here, airborne isolation should be instituted. All healthcare workers should wear N95 masks or other appropriate levels of protection when exposed to the patient and aerosol-producing procedures should be reduced if possible. Any suspected case of avian influenza should be reported to the institution's infection control service and local public health authorities immediately. Precautions should remain in place until deemed unnecessary by infection control and public health authorities.

Patient management

In order to make a prompt diagnosis, diagnostic specimens should be obtained as soon as possible. When avian influenza is suspected, pharyngeal swabs are the preferred specimen and reverse transcriptase–polymerase chain reaction (RT-PCR) assays are the rapid diagnostic method of choice. Isolation of H5N1 influenza viruses is time consuming and requires laboratory facilities of biosafety Level 3. Serological studies detecting H5N1-specific antibodies are not useful for rapid diagnostics, because specific antibodies are often not present early in disease. They remain important for diagnostic confirmation and epidemiological studies, however. The laboratory receiving specimens from cases of suspected avian influenza should be notified, in order to allow safe handling of specimens. In persons presenting with severe febrile respiratory illnesses of unknown aetiology, specimens should also be sent for investigation for bacterial and other viral pathogens.

The treatment of avian influenza is largely supportive with the addition of a neuraminidase inhibitor. Primary resistance against amantadine has been reported in some countries. The WHO advises the use of oseltamivir for the treatment of human H5N1 influenza infections. Efficacy of oseltamivir treatment is thought to be greater with earlier initiation. Little is actually known about its clinical effectiveness against human H5N1 infection, however, and antiviral treatment should not be withheld from persons presenting late. Antibacterial treatment guided by local epidemiology and epidemiology of the patient's travel destinations should also be commenced and continued until a definitive diagnosis is made.

Recent Developments

Oseltamivir-resistant H5N1 influenza virus has been reported and emergence of drug resistance may result in therapeutic failure. Combination antiviral therapy may be of benefit in this setting, such as a neuraminidase inhibitor with amantadine in cases where the virus remains amantadine susceptible. This requires further investigation. Alternatively, agents with targets other than neuraminidase or the M2 proton channel may be effective. Oseltamivir is currently available as an oral preparation. Parenteral formulations of neuraminidase inhibitors may result in more reliable therapeutic drug concentrations; such formulations are under development for zanamivir and peramivir. Many H5N1 vaccines have been experimentally tested and may, in the future, become important components of public health measures for pandemic control.

Conclusion

Febrile illnesses in travellers may represent emerging infectious diseases with pandemic potential. Although H5N1 influenza is not currently transmitted efficiently to humans, its high crude mortality when it does, and the potential for genomic mutation resulting in enhanced transmission, are reasons for increased attention to pandemic influenza preparation. Constant vigilance is required so that cases are promptly identified and appropriate infection control measures implemented in order to prevent secondary transmission. Appropriate specimens should be taken for rapid diagnostics. Treatment includes immediate commencement of oseltamivir as well as supportive measures. Public health authorities should be notified urgently in cases of suspected avian influenza infection.

Further Reading

Centers for Disease Control and Prevention. Interim guidance on planning for the use of surgical masks and respirators in health care settings during an influenza pandemic. Available at: http://www.flu.gov/professional/hospital/maskguidancehc.html (accessed 05 08 11).

Centers for Disease Control and Prevention. Respiratory hygiene/cough etiquette in healthcare settings. Available at: http://www.cdc.gov/flu/professionals/infectioncontrol/resphygiene.htm (accessed 05 08 11).

de Jong MD, Bach VC, Phan TQ *et al.* Fatal avian influenza A (H5N1) in a child presenting with diarrhea followed by coma. *N Engl J Med* 2005; **352**: 686–91.

Gambotto A, Barratt-Boyes SM, de Jong MD, Neumann G, Kawaoka Y. Human infection with highly pathogenic H5N1 influenza virus. *Lancet* 2008; **371**: 1464–75.

Harrod ME, Emery S, Dwyer DE. Antivirals in the management of an influenza pandemic. *Med J Aust* 2006; **185**(10 Suppl): S58–61.

Sandrock C, Stollenwerk N. Acute febrile respiratory illness in the ICU: reducing disease transmission. *Chest* 2008; **133**: 1221–31.

Schünemann HJ, Hill SR, Kakad M *et al.* WHO Rapid Advice Guidelines for pharmacological management of sporadic human infection with avian influenza A (H5N1) virus. *Lancet Infect Dis* 2007; **7**: 21–31.

World Health Organization. Affected areas with confirmed cases of H5N1 avian influenza. Available at: http://www.who.int/csr/disease/avian_influenza (accessed 05 08 11).

PROBLEM

45 Legionellosis

Dermot Kennedy

Case History

A 60-year-old diabetic smoker was air evacuated to the UK one week after admission to a hospital in Cancun, Mexico. He was referred following six days of fever, non-productive cough, diarrhoea and increasing confusion. Staying in a tourist hotel, he had briefly visited a rainforest. No pathogen was identified, he had not responded to intravenous co-amoxiclav, and four days post-admission right lung consolidation was noted. He then deteriorated despite substitution with meropenem and gentamicin.

On review he had a fever of 39.5°C, bilateral consolidation with pleural effusion, respiratory failure, early renal failure and gross hallucinosis. Investigations revealed microscopic haematuria, neutrophilia, hyponatraemia, mildly elevated serum bilirubin, transaminases and amylase, with a creatine kinase level of 12 500 U/l.

What are the most likely pathogens?

What diagnostic tests are most appropriate?

What treatment would you now initiate?

What complications should you be alert for?

Background

Travel may increase the risk of various respiratory infections including types common in the UK; those of lower UK prevalence such as Q fever and penicillin-resistant pneumococcus; and those non-endemic to the UK including tularaemia, H5N1 avian influenza and severe acute respiratory syndrome (SARS). Inquiry about geographical, lifestyle/leisure and other exposure is important, as is the type and/or degree of any underlying ill health.

Since in most cases of pneumonia no pathogen(s) is identified, therapy is invariably empirical. Distinguishing the type of pneumonia into a broad epidemiological category – e.g. community-, hospital-, travel-, immunosuppression- or influenza-related, or atypical – helps determine 'best guess' therapy, ideally compliant with local guidelines.

The atypical pneumonias are characterized by pronounced extrapulmonary features and non-response to β-lactam antibiotics, both evident in this case. Principal pathogens include *Mycoplasma pneumoniae*, *Chlamydia pneumoniae* and *C. psittaci*, *Legionella pneumophila* and *Coxiella burnetii*. Whilst not usually severe, some cases and certain pathogens, such as *C. psittaci* and *L. pneumophila*, may prove otherwise.

Discussion

Notable aspects of this case that have possible diagnostic/therapeutic implications include: prominent extrapulmonary features/complications; delayed recognition of severe pneumonia; potential exposure in a foreign hotel, hospital and tropical forest environment; and failure of broad antibiotic cover.

The diverse features and complications of this case suggest a severe atypical pneumonia, particularly Legionnaires' disease (LD) or psittacosis. The clinical pattern could also readily fit with pneumococcal pneumonia, notably bacteraemia with a penicillin-resistant organism or a nosocomial cause. A 'tropical' infection is unlikely, but typhoid fever or an exotic viral infection remain possibilities.

Prior antibiotic usage may compromise routine cultures of blood/sputum, which necessitates bronchoscopy in order to obtain specimens for microbiological culture and other diagnostic procedures. Tests for atypical organisms require serological, antigen or polymerase chain reaction (PCR) techniques. Timing is important here. For antigen or PCR tests, acute sampling is recommended, whereas serology may require two specimens over several weeks. Culture of Legionella requires special selective media but is the definitive, albeit slow, diagnostic method. Urinary antigen tests are increasingly employed, being rapid, highly specific, relatively sensitive and usable within three days before to several months after onset. Whilst only available for *L. pneumophila* serogroup 1, this accounts for about 80% of cases. Since no diagnostic method is entirely reliable, several should be employed.

The urgent requirement for this case is to provide cover against primarily 'atypical' pathogens. This requires antimicrobials with enhanced intracellular activity, given the intracellular sanctuary protecting these organisms from various antibiotics. Addressing specific aetiology, epidemiological clues, the unfolding clinical pattern, type of extrapulmonary manifestations and test results, the illness severity and its attendant pneumonia, and failure of β-lactam cover are certainly consistent with LD (Figure 45.1). Activity against Legionella is best provided by the newer macrolides, or rifampicin and/or quinolones.

The patient may harbour an antibiotic-resistant organism such as methicillin-resistant *Staphylococcus aureus* (MRSA) or a penicillin-resistant pneumococcus; these organisms would be covered by vancomycin.

Faced with his deterioration and a tangible possibility of LD, the optimum combination might be clarithromycin or levofloxacin with vancomycin, renal compromise necessitating dose modification of the latter. Several studies of LD suggest levofloxacin is superior to macrolides, but some would argue for a combination of these highly active drugs in severe/advanced LD. Assessment for intensive care should proceed urgently.

Urinary antigen testing now confirms the diagnosis of LD. Delay in initiating appropriate therapy has increased the risk of severe complications and death, which varies in the non-immunosuppressed from <1% to 13%. Respiratory failure requiring ventilation is the commonest of a diverse range of organ upset, and occurs in perhaps 20% of cases. Superinfection with another pathogen develops in about 10% of cases. Renal failure may intervene in severe disease but is usually reversible. Neurological complications range

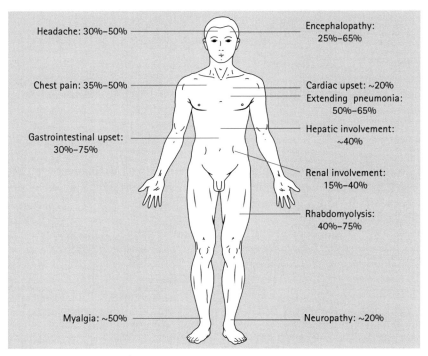

Figure 45.1 Aetiology of legionellosis.

from global encephalopathy to cerebellar damage, neuropathy and severe rhabdomyolysis. Damage from the latter sometimes proves longstanding. Indeed, fatigue, protracted over months or years, is common. Debate surrounds the frequency of extrapulmonary infection, but it often occurs in immunosuppression. Of various vulnerable organs, the heart seems most commonly affected, with endocarditis or myocarditis.

Further Considerations

Legionellosis exemplifies a modern paradigm of disease emergence grounded in the 'Triad of Infection'. The fortuitous conjunction of virulent pathogen, infection-enhancing environment and a susceptible, compromised host can culminate in lethal disease. Hence the physician must maintain a high index of suspicion for this protean, sometimes bewildering, condition to ensure adequate diagnosis and management. In its classic form, a constellation of clinico-investigational characteristics may strongly suggest a diagnosis of LD, yet studies have failed to identify any pathognomonic feature distinguishing it, in particular, from pneumococcal disease. All potentially severe pneumonias should be investigated using several methods to establish the diagnosis and receive empirical cover against legionellosis. LD ranks among the four most prominent community causes of pneumonia, not least when necessitating intensive care. This applies particularly if there is underlying disease, especially immunosuppression. A third of sporadic infections are linked with travel, where the association with man-made aquatic systems is clearly pertinent.

Conclusion

Cases of travel-associated pneumonia can pose various clinical challenges: management of unfamiliar or exotic conditions, problems in ascertaining prior care details, and the difficulties of presentation with advanced disease. For reasons involving both patient and public health, the advice of an infectious diseases specialist may be usefully sought.

Further Reading

Benin AL, Benson RF, Besser RE. Trends in Legionnaires disease, 1980–1998: declining mortality and new patterns of diagnosis. *Clin Infect Dis* 2002; **35**: 1039–46.

Blázques Garrido RM, Espinosa Parra FJ, Alemany Francés L *et al.* Antimicrobial chemotherapy for Legionnaires disease: levofloxacin versus macrolides. *Clin Infect Dis* 2005; **40**: 800–6.

Diederen BMW. *Legionella* spp. and Legionnaires' disease. *J Infect* 2008; **56**: 1–12.

Leder K, Sundararajan V, Weld L, Pandey P, Brown G, Torresi J. Respiratory tract infections in travelers: a review of the GeoSentinel surveillance network. *Clin Infect Dis* 2003; **36**: 399–406.

Sopena N, Sabrià-Leal M, Pedro-Botet ML *et al.* Comparative study of the clinical presentation of Legionella pneumonia and other community-acquired pneumonias. *Chest* 1998; **113**: 1195–2000.

HIV INFECTION

PROBLEM

46 HIV Seroconversion

Antonia Ho

Case History

A 29-year-old man was admitted with a week's history of general malaise accompanied by severe myalgia, abdominal pain, diarrhoea, headache, dry cough and swelling and redness of his eyes. He was a heavy drinker, and had fallen into the river Clyde two weeks previously while inebriated. On admission he was pyrexial (39.2°C) and tachycardic. Examination revealed conjunctival injection, sore red throat, cervical lymphadenopathy and a maculopapular rash on his trunk. He had deranged liver function (aspartate transaminase 770 IU/l, alanine transaminase 380 IU/l) and neutropenia.

He was initially treated with intravenous ceftriaxone, ciprofloxacin and metronidazole, with no improvement. Blood, stool and urine culture were negative. A subsequent test for Leptospira immunoglobulin M was negative, as was a viral hepatitis screen. Abdominal ultrasound showed mild splenomegaly. He disclosed an unprotected sexual contact from a month ago. His human immunodeficiency virus (HIV) antibody test returned positive. His baseline CD4 lymphocyte count was 580×10^6/l, with a viral load of 3 024 412 copies/ml.

What was the differential diagnosis of his presentation?

Would you consider antiretroviral therapy at this stage?

What is the prognosis of those presenting with HIV seroconversion illness?

Background

Given the constellation of symptoms and recent water contact, leptospirosis is an obvious differential diagnosis. Other possibilities are mononucleosis syndrome secondary to Epstein–Barr virus (EBV) or cytomegalovirus (CMV), viral hepatitis, streptococcal infection and toxoplasmosis. In fact, this patient has HIV seroconversion illness. He had a positive HIV antibody test, along with an extremely high viral load. His symptoms settled after two weeks. Three months after presentation, his CD4 lymphocyte count was 1117×10^6/l, with a dramatic fall in HIV-RNA to 154 copies/ml. The case illustrates the importance of a detailed social, and in particular, sexual history.

Primary HIV infection (PHI) describes the interval from initial infection to a detectable HIV antibody, characterized by a transient period of massive viral replication. It is a non-specific clinical syndrome that occurs two to four weeks after HIV exposure, but can occur at up to six months. The symptoms are self-limiting, lasting for an average of two weeks (Table 46.1). However, lymphadenopathy and fatigue may persist for months. Previous studies have suggested that duration and severity of symptoms predict a more rapid disease progression.

Table 46.1 Clinical features of primary HIV infection

Common	Less common
• Fever	• Hepatitis
• Rash	• Pancreatitis
• Fatigue	• Aseptic meningitis
• Sore throat	• Encephalopathy
• Generalized lymphadenopathy	
• Myalgia/arthralgia	
• Headache	
• Oral ulceration	
• Nausea/vomiting/diarrhoea	
• Weight loss	

Patients are highly infectious during this stage due to the markedly elevated viral load. It has been suggested that a large proportion of HIV infections may be transmitted by individuals with primary infection, though this remains controversial.

Rarely, opportunistic infections can occur during PHI. This is thought to be due to transient CD4 lymphopenia. Case reports of *Pneumocystis carinii* pneumonia, oral and oesophageal candidiasis, toxoplasmosis and CMV colitis have also been described.

Diagnosis

The diagnosis of PHI is demonstrated by a very high HIV-RNA (>100 000 copies/ml) and a negative or indeterminate HIV antibody in the context of risk exposure and typical clinical features. A false positive should be suspected if viral load is low (<1000 copies/ml). Patients with an indeterminate HIV antibody result and low viral loads should have repeat antibody testing in 4–6 weeks. Given the rising prevalence of transmitted HIV resistance, all patients with documented PHI should have a baseline resistance test.

PHI is underdiagnosed. The non-specific symptoms are often mistaken for influenza or mononucleosis syndrome. PHI can cause a false-positive heterophile antibody (monospot) test, with presence of atypical lymphocytes, making the differentiation between PHI and EBV infection even more difficult. Clinicians may be unaware of high-risk behaviour of their patients, or may feel uncomfortable broaching a sexual history. Additionally, those working in other fields who are unfamiliar with the clinical presentation may not even consider the diagnosis.

Treatment

The role of antiretroviral treatment in PHI is widely debated. It is unclear whether HIV progression can be altered by an immediate and time-limited therapeutic intervention. It is also not known whether initiation of therapy during PHI would yield greater benefits than initiating it later in the disease course (Table 46.2).

Table 46.2 HIV treatment: risks and benefits of early intervention

Potential benefits of early intervention:

- preserve immune function
- prevent viral diversification
- reduce risk of secondary transmission
- decrease severity of seroconversion illness

Risks of early intervention:

- drug toxicities from extended exposure to antiretroviral treatment
- development of resistance
- adherence issues in newly diagnosed patients
- cost implications
- viral rebound (cases of recurrent symptomatic PHI have been reported)

A number of observational studies investigating treatment during PHI have demonstrated limited, transient improvements in immunological outcomes. However, no study to date has addressed the role of antiretrovirals in PHI on long-term immunological, virological or clinical outcomes.

At present, routine initiation of antiretroviral treatment in PHI is not recommended, except in a clinical trial setting.

Recent Developments

SPARTAC is the first randomized controlled trial powered to determine the impact of limited treatment of PHI on the rate of CD4 cell decline, and therefore on time to initiation of clinically indicated antiretroviral therapy. It compares no intervention with treatment given for 12 or 48 weeks. Recruitment has been completed and the results are awaited.

Another ongoing randomized study (ACTG A5217) aims to address the virological outcome, comparing 36 weeks' treatment with tenofovir, emtricitabine and lopinavir/ritonavir against no therapy in PHI.

Conclusion

PHI is a non-specific syndrome that is poorly recognized. In patients presenting with a persistent, febrile, flu- or mononucleosis-like syndrome, risk factors for HIV infection should be ascertained including sexual activity, intravenous drug use and blood transfusion. A baseline HIV antibody test and viral load should be obtained.

Early diagnosis of PHI could be effective in reducing transmission. Given the public health implications, non-HIV/genitourinary medicine healthcare providers (especially in primary care) may benefit from training in case recognition to improve rates of diagnosis.

The definitive role of antiretroviral treatment in PHI remains unclear. Further clarification will await the results of ongoing clinical trials.

Further Reading

Acute Infection and Early Disease Research Program. ACTG A5217. A 96-week randomized, open-label study of the effects on virologic setpoint of 36 weeks of potent antiretroviral therapy administered during early but not acute HIV-1 infection. Available at: http://www.aiedrp.org/studies.asp (accessed 05 08 11).

Bell SK, Little SJ, Rosenberg ES. Clinical management of acute HIV infection: best practice remains unknown. *J Infect Dis* 2010; **202(Suppl 2)**: S278–88.

Fidler S, Fox J, Porter K, Weber J. Primary HIV infection: to treat or not to treat? *Curr Opin Infect Dis* 2008; **21**: 4–10.

Gazzard BG, Anderson J, Babiker *et al.*; BHIVA Treatment Guidelines Writing Group. British HIV Association Guidelines for the treatment of HIV-1-infected adults with antiretroviral therapy 2008. *HIV Med* 2008; **9**: 563–608.

Medical Research Council Clinical Trials Unit. Short pulse anti-retroviral therapy at seroconversion (SPARTAC). MRC, 2006. Available at: http://www.ctu.mrc.ac.uk/research_areas/study_details.aspx?s=32 (accessed 05 08 11).

Pilcher CD, Tien HC, Eron JJ Jr *et al*. Brief but efficient: acute HIV infection and the sexual transmission of HIV. *J Infect Dis* 2004; **189**: 1785–92.

Vanhems P, Lambert J, Cooper DA *et al*. Severity and prognosis of acute human immunodeficiency virus type 1 illness: a dose-response relationship. *Clin Infect Dis* 1998; **26**: 323–9.

47 Cryptococcal Disease in HIV

Neil D. Ritchie

Case History

A 43-year-old Zimbabwean woman presented with headache and meningism of several weeks' duration. A computed tomography (CT) scan of the brain was normal but lumbar puncture revealed an elevated opening pressure and lymphocytic cerebrospinal fluid (CSF) with encapsulated yeasts seen on India ink staining. *Cryptococcus neoformans* was subsequently cultured from blood and CSF. A human immunodeficiency virus (HIV) test was positive with a CD4 lymphocyte count of 9×10^6/l. She was treated with antifungals, and highly active antiretroviral therapy (HAART) was introduced after four weeks, but despite this she continued to have symptoms of raised intracranial pressure for several months, despite repeated lumbar puncture. Her symptoms acutely worsened around two months into her treatment. She now had haemorrhagic papilloedema and an abducens nerve palsy.

What is the optimum antifungal management of cryptococcal meningitis?

How should her raised intracranial pressure be managed?

What is the optimum time to introduce HAART?

Background

Cryptococcal disease is a common opportunistic infection in patients with immuno-suppression secondary to HIV infection. In southern Africa it is now the most commonly identified cause of meningitis, reflecting the high prevalence of HIV infection in those countries. In the developed world, cryptococcal meningitis has become less common since the introduction of HAART but remains a problem in those presenting with advanced HIV infection. The majority of patients have CD4 lymphocyte counts of $<50 \times 10^6$/l and it is rare in patients with CD4 lymphocyte counts $>100 \times 10^6$/l.

The presentation of cryptococcal meningitis is usually insidious with several weeks of headache, meningism and fever. Visual disturbance and altered conscious level are late signs. Since early central nervous system infection can present with vague symptoms in patients with low CD4 lymphocyte counts, clinicians should maintain a high index of suspicion. Investigation is with CT scanning of the brain followed by lumbar puncture. Since raised intracranial pressure is usually not visible on imaging studies and has significant implications on management, quantification of the opening pressure is mandatory. India ink staining of the CSF will demonstrate cryptococci in around 70% of cases. Alternatively, detection of cryptococcal polysaccharide antigen in CSF or blood is highly sensitive, while Cryptococcus can usually be cultured from CSF and blood.

Antifungal therapy

Management of cryptococcal meningitis has been the subject of several randomized controlled trials, and treatment guidelines exist. A treatment algorithm is shown in Figure 47.1. The combination of amphotericin B with flucytosine is the most effective initial therapy and is generally accepted as the optimum treatment. This initial therapy is usually given for two weeks before the substitution of azole monotherapy, usually with high-dose fluconazole for eight weeks. Once ten weeks of therapy is completed, the patient should be treated with long-term suppressive therapy usually consisting of azole monotherapy at a lower dose. Current treatment guidelines suggest that this therapy be continued indefinitely but a more recent randomized controlled trial suggests that patients established on HAART with a CD4 lymphocyte count $>100 \times 10^6$/l, an undetectable viral load and negative cryptococcal antigen can safely discontinue this therapy.

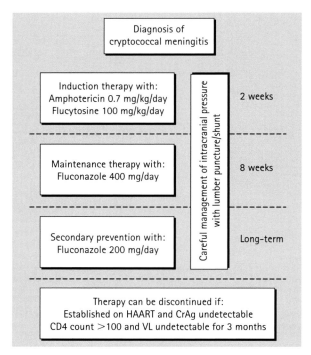

Figure 47.1 Treatment algorithm for the management of cryptococcal meningitis. CrAg, cryptococcal antigen; HAART, highly active antiretroviral therapy; VL, viral load.

Raised intracranial pressure

A major cause of morbidity and mortality in cryptococcal meningitis is elevated intracranial pressure. This usually occurs without the development of hydrocephalus. Failure to aggressively manage elevated intracranial pressure has been associated with poor clinical outcome. Serial lumbar puncture, with the removal of 20–30 ml of CSF on each occasion, is frequently required to reduce the intracranial pressure. Sometimes, as in our patient's case, frequent lumbar puncture was insufficient to control intracranial pressure. In this case, a neurosurgeon was consulted and an Ommaya reservoir (a ventricular drain implanted subcutaneously over the vault of the skull) was inserted, which allowed the serial removal of larger amounts of CSF. Alternatives include insertion of lumbar drains or ventriculoperitoneal shunts. There is no evidence that pharmacological options are effective for the management of raised intracranial pressure and both corticosteroids and acetazolamide have been associated with poorer outcomes.

Recent Developments

The optimal timing of antiretroviral therapy remains a subject of active investigation. Conventionally, antiretroviral therapy has been delayed in patients presenting with opportunistic infection. This is due to concern about potential drug interactions, drug absorption in acutely unwell patients and the risk of immune reconstitution inflammatory syndrome (IRIS). The acute deterioration in our patient's condition most likely represented this latter complication, since there was no evidence of microbiological failure of therapy. However, recent evidence suggests that early initiation of antiretroviral therapy is beneficial for patients with opportunistic infection.

In a randomized, open-label study, patients presenting with opportunistic infection treated with immediate HAART fared better in a composite end-point of death and acquired immune deficiency syndrome progression compared to patients in whom treatment was deferred. However, the study included only 35 patients with cryptococcal meningitis and while the trend in those patients was similar, the small numbers preclude definite conclusions. Further work is required to provide more precise information on when to give patients with cryptococcal meningitis HAART.

Another important area of ongoing research is the IRIS associated with cryptococcal meningitis. This is a paradoxical worsening of symptoms despite successful antimicrobial management in temporal association with commencing HAART; this includes recurrence of fever, meningism or raised intracranial pressure. IRIS is thought to occur in around 10%–15% of patients. However, evidence thus far is based on small studies and treatment remains undefined, although steroids have been used with apparent success in case reports. More work is needed to guide investigation and management of cryptococcal IRIS, particularly since it may become more frequent as HAART is introduced earlier in the course of treatment.

Conclusion

Worldwide, cryptococcal meningitis is the commonest neurological complication of HIV infection. Prior to the advent of antiretroviral therapy, this complication was universally fatal. Modern-day management is complicated and requires expert clinical care with regard to drug-related toxicity, drug–drug interactions (particularly between the azole antifungals and antiretroviral therapy), raised intracranial pressure and the potentially life-threatening IRIS. Despite these challenges, long-term outcome in HIV-related cryptococcal meningitis is now excellent.

Further Reading

Graybill JR, Sobel J, Saag M *et al*. Diagnosis and management of increased intracranial pressure in patients with AIDS and cryptococcal meningitis. The NIAID Mycoses Study Group and AIDS Cooperative Treatment Groups. *Clin Infect Dis* 2000; **30**: 47–54.

Lodha A, Haran M. Is it recurrent cryptococcal meningitis or immune reconstitution inflammatory syndrome? *Int J STD AIDS* 2009; **20**: 666–7.

Perfect JR, Dismukes WE, Dromer F *et al*. Clinical Practice Guidelines for the Management of Cryptococcal Disease: 2010 Update by the Infectious Diseases Society of America. *Clin Infect Dis* 2010; **50**: 291–322.

Sungkanuparph S, Filler SG, Chetchotisakd P *et al*. Cryptococcal immune reconstitution inflammatory syndrome after antiretroviral therapy in AIDS patients with cryptococcal meningitis: a prospective multicenter study. *Clin Infect Dis* 2009; **49**: 931–4.

Vibhagool A, Sungkanuparph S, Mootsikapun P *et al*. Discontinuation of secondary prophylaxis for cryptococcal meningitis in human immunodeficiency virus-infected patients treated with highly active antiretroviral therapy: a prospective, multicenter, randomized study. *Clin Infect Dis* 2003; **36**: 1329–31.

Zolopa A, Andersen J, Powderly W *et al*. Early antiretroviral therapy reduces AIDS progression/death in individuals with acute opportunistic infections: a multicenter randomized strategy trial. *PLoS One* 2009; **4**: e5575.

PROBLEM

48 *Pneumocystis jirovecii* Pneumonia

Alec Bonington

Case History

A 55-year-old man presented with a four-week history of dry cough and fever. He had become progressively more short of breath over the previous seven days. On examination, he appeared dyspnoeic at rest. He was thin and demonstrated both oropharyngeal candidiasis and oral hairy leukoplakia. Auscultation of the lung fields was clear. He disclosed no risk factors for human immunodeficiency virus (HIV) infection although he had previously worked extensively in West Africa in the oil industry. He reported a negative HIV test (for insurance purposes) five years previously. He had presented to the local emergency department a week previously, when a chest X-ray was performed, appeared normal and had been sent home with a seven-day course of amoxicillin, but he had continued to deteriorate. On admission, respiratory rate was 24 breaths/min, oxygen saturation on air was 91% and chest X-ray was abnormal (Figure 48.1).

What are the important factors to elicit in the history?

Which diagnostic tests are essential?

What should the management strategy be?

What is the optimum time to commence antiretroviral therapy?

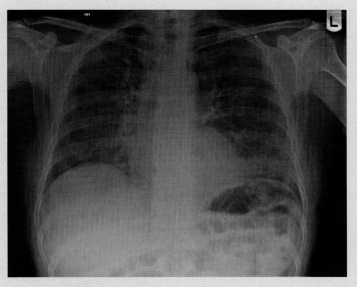

Figure 48.1 Chest X-ray of *Pneumocystis jirovecii* pneumonia demonstrating extensive bilateral interstitial infiltrates.

Background

Pneumocystis jirovecii pneumonia (PCP) is the commonest acquired immune deficiency syndrome (AIDS)-defining illness seen in the UK. As in this case, it typically has an insidious onset and is often the presenting illness of HIV infection. PCP should therefore be considered in any patient with a respiratory illness of insidious onset. It is important to establish risk factors for HIV infection by ascertaining a detailed sexual history, history of injecting drug use, and a detailed travel history, including country of origin, given the higher prevalence of HIV in certain parts of the world such as sub-Saharan Africa, India and Southeast Asia. In this case, risk factors (heterosexual contacts in West Africa) were not immediately appreciated or volunteered by the patient. An HIV antibody test should be offered if any risk factors for HIV are present, when a presenting illness is compatible with a complication of HIV or HIV enters the differential diagnosis. In patients infected with HIV, the CD4 lymphocyte count (normal range 500–1500 × 10⁶/l) is a guide to the level of immunosuppression and which opportunistic infections such a patient may be at risk of developing. PCP is unlikely to develop in those with a CD4 lymphocyte count in excess of $200 \times 10^6/l$.

With current antiretroviral therapy (ART), the prognosis following successful treatment of PCP is excellent. It is important to remember that PCP can occur in non-HIV immunocompromised patients (particularly those not receiving PCP prophylaxis) too. These include patients taking steroids, methotrexate, cyclophosphamide and anti–tumour necrosis factor agents. The presentation of PCP in this group of patients tends to be much more rapid (several days rather than a few weeks) than those infected with HIV. Investigation of suspected PCP is summarized in Table 48.1.

Table 48.1 Summary of investigation of a patient with suspected PCP

HIV testing. Mandatory in all patients in whom HIV status is not known.

Exercise oximetry – a bedside test where oxygen saturations are performed at rest on air and then after exercise such as walking up a flight of stairs. A significant reduction after exercise suggests PCP in someone with a normal or near-normal chest X-ray. Remember, resting oxygen saturations may be normal in early disease.

Chest X-ray – this may be normal in 10% or more of patients at presentation, as in the case described when he first presented. Bilateral perihilar shadowing tends to be the earliest radiological abnormality. Lung cysts are also sometimes seen and diffuse bilateral shadowing can occur in late disease.

Induced sputum samples for PCP PCR. This has the highest sensitivity for the diagnosis of PCP although false positives are recognized.

Arterial blood gases on air where the oxygen saturations are reduced. This helps to determine the need for adjunctive steroid therapy (see 'Treatment' in main text).

PCR, polymerase chain reaction.

Treatment

Delay in treatment can be catastrophic so patients with an appropriate history, reduction in oxygen saturation on exercise and a chest X-ray compatible with PCP (including normal chest X-ray) should be commenced on empirical therapy. Attempts to confirm the diagnosis should then be made as above.

First-line therapy for PCP consists of high-dose co-trimoxazole at a dose of 120 mg/kg in 3–4 divided doses for three weeks. This is given orally in mild cases but should be given intravenously (IV), at least initially, in more severe cases. Mortality is reduced when steroids are given in those patients with an oxygen pressure (pO_2) on air of <9.3 kPa. It is not uncommon for the patient to deteriorate and become more hypoxic around day four of treatment. However, if the patient continues to deteriorate after day seven, treatment failure needs to be considered and second-line therapy instituted. Furthermore, many patients are unable to tolerate co-trimoxazole due to allergy or other side effects and need to be switched to second-line treatment.

Optimal second-line treatment is a combination of clindamycin IV (600 mg every 8 hours) and primaquine (30 mg daily). It is essential to exclude glucose 6-phosphate dehydrogenase (G6PD) deficiency before commencing this regimen as severe haemolysis can occur when primaquine is given to G6PD-deficient individuals. Physicians using this regime also need to be vigilant for methaemoglobinaemia, secondary to primaquine. For severe disease, another alternative is pentamidine IV. Oral atovaquone at a dose of 750 mg bd may be used as an alternative for mild to moderate disease. There is an increased risk of pneumothorax in PCP and this should be considered if the patient becomes suddenly more dyspnoeic or develops pleuritic chest pain. After completion of treatment for PCP, prophylaxis against this pathogen needs to be continued until the CD4 lymphocyte count exceeds 200×10^6/l.

Recent Developments

One of the big uncertainties when managing HIV-positive patients with PCP and other opportunistic infections (OI) has always been when to commence ART. Concern has been fuelled by observations of rapid deterioration following commencement of ART, potentially driven by a brisk immune reconstitution inflammatory syndrome. The ACTG 5164 study randomized HIV-positive patients with OI (PCP 63%, cryptococcal meningitis 12%, bacterial infection 12%) to either commence early ART (within 14 days of starting treatment for their OI) or defer ART until after completing treatment for their OI. In this study, those receiving early ART had a significant reduction in AIDS progression and/or death compared to the deferred arm. A prerequisite for this study was that patients had to be able to take oral therapy, so potentially excluding critically unwell patients. Results therefore need to be interpreted carefully and case-by-case judgement is required particularly in the critically ill patients unable to take oral therapy. Furthermore, optimal timing of commencement of ART in those able to take oral therapy within the first two weeks remains uncertain.

Conclusion

Pneumocystis jirovecii should always be considered in HIV-positive patients with respiratory tract infections. With current antiretroviral therapy, the prognosis following successful treatment of PCP is excellent.

Further Reading

Briel M, Bucher H, Boscacci R, Furrer H. Adjunctive corticosteroids for *Pneumocystis jiroveci* pneumonia in patients with HIV-infection. *Cochrane Database Syst Rev* 2006; CD006150. DOI: 10.1002/14651858.CD006150.

Catherinot E, Lanternier F, Bougnoux M-E, Lecuit M, Couderc LJ, Lortholary O. *Pneumocystis jirovecii* pneumonia. *Infect Dis Clin North Am* 2010; **24**: 107–38.

Zolopa AR, Andersen J, Powderly W *et al.* Early antiretroviral therapy reduces AIDS progression/ death in individuals with acute opportunistic infections: a multicenter randomized strategy trial. *PLoS One* 2009; **4**: e5575.

PROBLEM

49 Needlestick Injuries and Post-exposure Prophylaxis Against HIV Infection

Nneka Nwokolo

Case History

A junior doctor is referred by the occupational health department having sustained a deep puncture wound to his left thumb 30 minutes previously. He had been attempting to resheath an arterial blood gas needle used on an unconscious patient admitted the day before with *Pneumocystis jirovecii* pneumonia. The patient was a Kenyan male aged 28 years and was accompanied by his elder brother. He had recently come to the UK having been unwell for several weeks with fevers, weight loss and increasing shortness of breath. His human immunodeficiency virus (HIV) status was unknown.

What data are there on the efficacy of HIV post-exposure prophylaxis (PEP) following needlestick injury or mucosal exposure?

What are the indications for PEP?

What are the legalities regarding the testing of patients unable to give consent?

What should be considered when deciding which PEP regimen to prescribe?

What other infections should be considered following a needlestick injury?

Background

The risk of transmission following a needlestick injury involving a known HIV-positive source is about 0.3%, while that following mucosal (e.g. blood splash to mucous membrane or non-intact skin) injury is approximately 0.1%.

This risk may be reduced by administration of antiretroviral therapy as soon as possible after injury (ideally within 1 hour and certainly within 72 hours). This is known as post-exposure prophylaxis or PEP.

A retrospective case–control study of healthcare workers exposed to HIV infection demonstrated an 81% reduction in transmission in individuals given PEP with zidovudine (AZT) compared to individuals not receiving PEP (Cardo *et al.*, 1997). Animal data and mother-to-child transmission studies also demonstrate the efficacy of PEP. Mathematical modelling shows that the reduction in transmission seen in babies born to HIV-positive women receiving antiretroviral therapy immediately prior to delivery occurs as a result of PEP.

Management of individuals exposed to HIV infection

Following a needlestick injury, immediate first-aid measures should be performed (Figure 49.1). Consideration of the nature and degree of injury, as well as the knowledge or likelihood that the source patient (i.e. the individual from whom the injury was received) is HIV-positive, is warranted.

Factors associated with increased risk of transmission include the prior presence of the needle in a blood vessel; deep injury; injury with a hollow needle; and terminal disease in the source patient (where the patient is not on treatment and has a high viral load). Exposure of intact skin to HIV-infected blood is not considered significant.

To reduce anxiety in the injured healthcare worker and to prevent unnecessary prescription of drugs known to have significant side effects and unknown long-term toxicity, efforts should be made to establish the presence of infection where the status of the source is unknown. A risk assessment should be performed to ascertain the likelihood of the source individual being HIV-positive. This should take into account such factors as the age, prevalence of HIV in the country of origin and sexual orientation (higher prevalence of HIV infection in homosexual men than in heterosexual men in the UK). The UK Department of Health, however, advocates a universal approach to source-patient testing in order to avoid potential discrimination against groups perceived to be at high risk of infection.

Source-patient testing should be performed as soon as possible, but only after a pretest discussion covering the relevant issues relating to HIV transmission. Informed consent to disclose the test results to the healthcare worker concerned and the occupational health service should be obtained. Pre-test discussion should not be performed by the injured healthcare worker, but may be performed by any other trained member of the healthcare team. Where testing of the source patient is not immediately possible, PEP may be initiated while attempts are made to obtain consent.

It is against the law for HIV testing to be performed without consent unless it is deemed to be in the patient's best interests. Testing must not be performed solely for the benefit of the affected healthcare worker. The General Medical Council recommends that where it is not possible to obtain consent, legal advice as well as guidance from local occupational health staff should be sought.

If an injury is considered significant and the source patient is known to be, or highly likely to be, HIV-positive, treatment should be administered as soon as possible for 28 days with any of the standard antiretroviral regimens recommended for PEP. Most hospitals in the UK have local guidance on which drugs to use and the Department of Health document referred to above is also helpful. Individuals for whom PEP is prescribed should be followed-up by a physician experienced in the management of HIV-infected patients.

A regimen consisting of three antiretroviral drugs is recommended in the UK, although there are no data to demonstrate the superiority of this over monotherapy. The rationale for this is based on the fact that at least three drugs are necessary to control infection in HIV-positive individuals. Until recently, most PEP regimens included AZT as this is the only drug for which there are efficacy data. However, AZT is associated with significant short-term toxicity and many people who take it are unable to complete the four-week course. Most guidelines have now replaced AZT with drugs causing fewer side

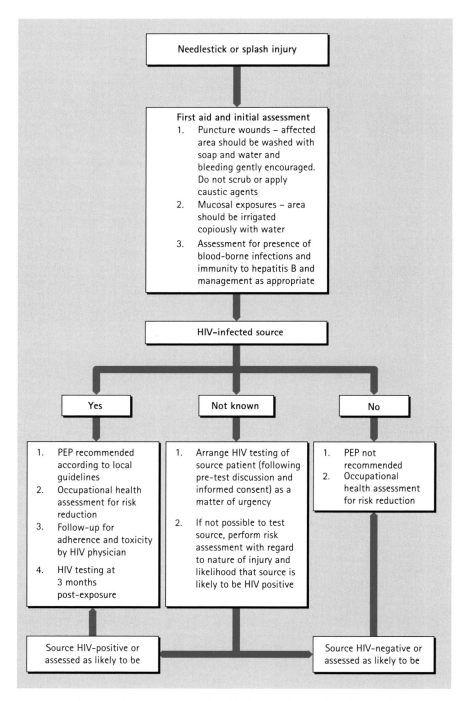

Figure 49.1 Algorithm for management of individuals sustaining needlestick or splash injury.

effects. A commonly advocated regimen with relatively low toxicity is tenofovir 245 mg daily, emtricitabine 200 mg daily and 400 mg lopinavir/100 mg ritonavir combination twice daily. Choice of regimen should be influenced by knowledge of current or previous treatment of the source patient, toxicity and information about possible antiretroviral resistance.

The junior doctor described in this case sustained a significant injury from a patient of unknown HIV status who was at high risk of HIV infection and likely to have a high viral load (having presented with advanced disease). PEP would be strongly recommended and treatment with the lopinavir/ritonavir-based regimen described above would be appropriate.

Exposure to other blood-borne pathogens including hepatitis B and hepatitis C should also be considered in any healthcare worker sustaining a needlestick injury. Clinical staff should ensure that they are vaccinated against hepatitis B and vaccination should be offered to unvaccinated individuals. There is no vaccination or prophylaxis against hepatitis C so early identification and treatment of infected individuals is required and has been shown to reduce the risk of developing chronic infection.

It is crucial that practices which increase the risk of needlestick injuries (e.g. resheathing of needles) are identified and corrected. Healthcare workers who sustain these injuries should be assessed by occupational health staff and encouraged to modify their practices if necessary.

Recent Developments

Recent data suggest that the risk of sexual transmission of HIV from individuals with a viral load below 50 copies/ml is extremely low. It is likely that this is also the case following needlestick injury but there are currently no data to support this.

PEP is also now routinely recommended following sexual exposure to HIV infection after unprotected intercourse. HIV-discordant couples particularly should be counselled on this aspect of care.

Conclusion

HIV PEP should be considered in the event of any significant exposure to body fluids in a healthcare worker. PEP is highly effective in reducing the transmission of HIV infection and the availability of antiretroviral drugs with fewer side effects means that PEP regimens can now be constructed that enable easier completion of treatment.

Further Reading

Cardo DM, Culver DH, Ciesielski CA *et al*. A case-control study of HIV seroconversion in health care workers after percutaneous exposure. *New Engl J Med* 1997; **337**: 1485–90.

Connor EM, Sperling RS, Gelber R *et al*. Reduction of maternal-infant transmission of human immunodeficiency virus type 1 with zidovudine treatment. *New Engl J Med* 1994; **331**: 1173–80.

Department of Health, UK. HIV post-exposure prophylaxis: guidance from the UK Chief Medical Officers' Expert Advisory Group on AIDS. UK Department of Health, 2008. Available at: http://

www.dh.gov.uk/en/Publicationsandstatistics/Publications/PublicationsPolicyAndGuidance/DH_088185 (accessed 05 08 11).

General Medical Council. Serious communicable diseases. Available at: http://www.gmc-uk.org/guidance/serious_communicable_diseases/index.asp (accessed 05 08 11).

Nwokolo NC, Barton S. Sharps injuries. *Care Critically Ill* 2002; **18**: 187–91.

Raphael J. Landovitz, RJ, Currier JS. Postexposure prophylaxis for HIV infection. *N Engl J Med* 2009; **361**: 1768–75.

Tsai EC, Emau P, Follis K *et al.* Effectiveness of postinoculation (R)-9-(2-phosphonylmethoxy-propyl) adenine treatment for prevention of persistent simian immunodeficiency virus SIV$_{mne}$ infection depends critically on timing of initiation and duration of treatment. *J Virol* 1998; **72**: 4265–73.

Wilson DP, Law MG, Grulich A, Cooper DA, Kaldor JM. Relationship between HIV viral load and infectiousness: a model-based analysis. *Lancet* 2008; **372**: 314–20.

INFECTIONS IN DRUG USERS

PROBLEM

50 Jaundice in an Injecting Drug User

Alexander Mackenzie

Case History

A 28-year-old unemployed injecting drug user was admitted with a ten-day history of lethargy, malaise, nausea, upper abdominal discomfort and fever. Despite improvement in these symptoms, he had noticed yellowness of his eyes and skin over the past three days. Three years previously he had been diagnosed with chronic hepatitis C virus (HCV) infection when he had tested HCV antibody-positive and HCV RNA (polymerase chain reaction [PCR])-positive (genotype 3). Treatment had not been offered due to a chaotic lifestyle. Immunization against hepatitis A and hepatitis B had been declined. Other past medical history included injection-related groin abscesses, bilateral ilio-femoral deep venous thromboses and overdoses with heroin. He smoked tobacco and cannabis, but denied drinking alcohol. On examination he was icteric with a palpable liver edge but no stigmata of chronic liver disease or hepatic encephalopathy. Blood results are shown in Table 50.1.

What is the likely cause of his jaundice?

What is the prognosis?

How should he be treated?

Could this illness have been prevented?

Table 50.1 Blood results	
Test	Result (normal range)
Bilirubin	112 µmol/l (1–22)
Alanine aminotransferase	916 U/l (5–35)
Alkaline phosphatase	398 U/l (45–105)
Gamma glutamyl transferase	315 U/l (<50)
Hepatitis A IgM antibody	Negative
Hepatitis A total antibody	Negative
Hepatitis B surface antigen (HBsAg)	Positive
Hepatitis B core IgM antibody	Positive
Hepatitis B e antigen	Positive
Hepatitis B e antibody	Negative
Hepatitis C RNA (PCR)	Positive
Hepatitis D antigen and antibody	Negative
HIV antibody	Negative
HIV, human immunodeficiency virus; IgM, immunoglobulin M.	

Background

There is currently an injecting drug use (IDU) epidemic affecting most developed countries. Heroin use is common, although cocaine, amphetamine and benzodiazepine use is also prevalent. IDU has many potential medical complications including overdose, venous thrombosis, pulmonary thromboembolism, arterial occlusion, chemical injury and local or systemic bacterial infection. Psychiatric disorders, especially depression, and social problems such as family breakdown, criminal activity and imprisonment often follow.

The nature of the hepatic injury and jaundice in this case is suggested by the marked transaminitis indicating an acute hepatitis. Haemolytic anaemia, decompensated chronic liver disease, liver metastases or biliary obstruction will present different biochemical abnormalities. While acute hepatitis B is the commonest cause of acute hepatitis in IDU, other viruses, such as Epstein–Barr virus and cytomegalovirus, may also cause hepatitis but seldom jaundice. There are many other causes of acute hepatitis, particularly drugs such as alcohol, paracetamol and Ecstasy. The possibility of pre-existing liver disease, e.g. alcoholic liver disease, autoimmune liver disease, haemochromatosis, Wilson's disease, and hepatoma, should not be overlooked.

Positive hepatitis B core immunoglobulin M antibody indicates acute hepatitis B virus (HBV) infection. Chronic hepatitis C with active viral replication is evident as indicated by positive HCV RNA PCR. He has neither acute hepatitis A virus (HAV) infection nor HAV immunity through previous infection or vaccination.

Acute hepatitis and IDU

In drug users hepatitis B usually results from the sharing of injecting paraphernalia and several large outbreaks in drug-using communities have been observed. In the UK, IDU is associated with a 17% risk of HBV infection. Sexual transmission of HBV in this population is less common. There have also been IDU-related outbreaks of HAV, probably relating to poor standards of sanitation rather than transmission through sharing injection materials.

More than 95% of patients with acute HBV infection eliminate infection, with loss of hepatitis B surface antigen (HBsAg) and the development of hepatitis B surface antibodies. Given a good prognosis for acute hepatitis B, antiviral therapy is not usually indicated. A minority do develop fulminant liver failure, however, so careful follow-up is required, looking for features of encephalopathy or impaired 'hepatic' synthetic function (falling albumin and prolonged prothrombin time). Rarely, fulminant acute hepatitis B, manifesting as liver failure, may require liver transplantation.

Chronic hepatitis B (CHB) is defined as the presence of HBsAg for more than six months. The risk of CHB is related to the age at acute infection, being much more common in those infected in infancy and childhood.

Chronic hepatitis C and IDU

IDU in the UK is associated with about 50% HCV antibody positivity. The diagnosis is usually made through opportunistic screening due to current or previous risk behaviour or investigation of abnormal liver enzymes. Fewer than 20% of hepatitis C diagnoses are made during the acute illness. There is an increasing emphasis on 'case finding' of patients with undiagnosed chronic HCV infection so that treatment may be offered in order to reduce the risk of long-term complications.

The patient described had evidence of chronic hepatitis C, with the presence of RNA confirming viral replication. Assuming he makes a good recovery from the acute hepatitis B, consideration should be given to the management of his chronic hepatitis C. He should be offered help to stop using drugs, and given advice on how to avoid transmission of HCV and healthy lifestyle measures, including minimizing alcohol intake if relevant.

Guidance on treatment with pegylated interferon (PEG-INF) and ribavirin has been available for several years (e.g. Scottish Intercollegiate Guidelines Network, Guideline Number 92).

Chronic hepatitis B and hepatitis C co-infection

Compared with HCV mono-infection, HBV/HCV co-infected patients tend to have more severe liver injury, a higher probability of cirrhosis, hepatic decompensation and hepatocellular carcinoma. For those with dominant HCV infection and low-level HBV viraemia, treatment with PEG-INF and ribavirin can be as effective as in HCV mono-infection. For co-infected patients with dually active HBV and HCV, the optimal regimen for therapy is unclear, although adding oral nucleos(t)ide analogues (to treat HBV) to PEG-INF and ribavirin has been suggested.

Co-infection with HIV and hepatitis B or hepatitis C

In the UK, IDU has a low risk of human immunodeficiency virus (HIV) infection (0.7%–1.5%) and this patient tested HIV antibody-negative. Co-infection with HIV is associated with a more progressive natural history and worse response to treatment for both chronic hepatitis B and hepatitis C. The updated British HIV Association guidelines are recommended for further information on management.

Co-infection with hepatitis D (Delta virus infection)

Hepatitis Delta virus (HDV) infection is uncommon in the UK. An incomplete RNA virus, it requires HBV for its survival and replication. It is mainly associated with IDU, sexual partners and female sex workers. This patient has no evidence of HDV infection but it should be suspected if the acute hepatitis B is severe or if a patient with chronic hepatitis B develops acute hepatitis (superinfection). There is a high rate of fulminant hepatitis and progression to cirrhosis. The response to treatment is poor. HDV infection is preventable by HBV immunization.

Public health issues

IDU is an indication for HBV, HCV and HIV testing. In non-immune patients HBV and HAV immunization should be offered. An accelerated schedule of HBV vaccination (doses at 0, 1, 2 and 12 months) is recommended for high-risk groups where rapid protection is required. Household and sexual contacts of those with acute or chronic hepatitis B should also be offered testing and immunization against HBV as it is easily transmitted through blood or body fluids. Advice on how to reduce the risk of transmission of blood-borne viruses and how to minimize other injection-related risks is also important.

Recent Developments

Reactivation of hepatitis B

Most patients make a good clinical recovery from acute HBV infection and become HBsAg-negative. However, as HBV DNA persists in hepatocytes patients are at risk of HBV reactivation if they become immunodeficient (e.g. due to advanced HIV infection or organ transplantation) or are treated with chemotherapy or immunomodulatory drugs such as adalimumab, certolizumab, etanercept, infliximab or rituximab. Careful monitoring of liver function tests and for HBV reactivation is required. All patients considered for immunosuppressive therapy should be tested for evidence of previous hepatitis B infection by testing for HBV core total antibody, as well as HBsAg.

New drugs for chronic hepatitis B

The treatment of chronic hepatitis B is an evolving and difficult area, not least because of the lack of agreement on how to judge success, but also because of the increasing range of treatment options. Lamivudine is no longer recommended because of the development of resistance. The following drugs have been recommended by the UK National Institute for Health and Clinical Excellence (NICE) for treatment of chronic hepatitis B (in the absence of hepatitis C, hepatitis D and HIV): adefovir, peginterferon alfa-2a, entecavir and tenofovir. At the time of writing, NICE is undertaking an appraisal of entecavir and tenofovir for the treatment of chronic hepatitis B in adults with decompensated liver disease.

New drugs for chronic hepatitis C

Improved understanding of the HCV life cycle has led to the development of new types of antiviral therapy. Protease inhibitors, e.g. telaprevir and boceprevir, are due to be marketed in 2011. They have high antiviral activity, but monotherapy is associated with frequent selection of resistance. The addition of a protease inhibitor to PEG-INF and ribavirin substantially improves sustained virological response rates and it is expected that protease inhibitors will be used in triple combination regimens. A number of polymerase inhibitors, which have a higher genetic barrier to resistance, are expected to reach the market by 2015. Patients may then be treated with an interferon-sparing triple regimen (polymerase inhibitor, protease inhibitor and ribavirin) or a more expensive quadruple therapy regimen.

Conclusion

- Determining the cause of jaundice in IDU is usually relatively straightforward but causes other than viral hepatitis should be considered.
- The prognosis of acute hepatitis B in IDU is usually good with a small risk of chronic hepatitis B.
- Patients with previous hepatitis B infection are at risk of reactivation if they become immunocompromised due to disease or treatment.
- Guidelines for the management of chronic hepatitis B and hepatitis C continue to evolve as our understanding of the natural history improves and new treatments become available.
- The introduction of a range of new therapeutic agents is likely to transform the treatment of chronic hepatitis C in the coming years.

Acknowledgement

The author thanks Dr Pamela Molyneaux for reviewing the manuscript.

Further Reading

Brook G, Main J, Nelson M *et al*. British HIV Association guidelines for the management of coinfection with HIV-1 and hepatitis B or C virus 2010. *HIV Med* 2010; **11**:1–30.

Chu CJ, Lee SD. Hepatitis B virus/hepatitis C virus coinfection: epidemiology, clinical features, viral interactions and treatment. *J Gastroenterol Hepatol* 2008; **23**: 512–20.

European Association For The Study Of The Liver. EASL Clinical Practice Guidelines: management of chronic hepatitis B. *J Hepatol* 2009; **50**: 227–42.

Health Protection Agency. Shooting Up. Infections among injecting drug users in the UK 2009. London: Health Protection Agency, 2010. Available at: http://www.hpa.org.uk/web/HPAwebFile/HPAweb_C/1287143384395 (accessed 05 08 11).

Scottish Intercollegiate Guidelines Network (SIGN). Management of hepatitis C. A national clinical guideline. Guideline No. 92. Edinburgh: SIGN, 2006. Available at: http://www.sign.ac.uk/pdf/sign92.pdf (accessed 01 09 11).

Vermehren J, Sarrazin C. New HCV therapies on the horizon. *Clin Microbiol Infect* 2011; **17**: 122–34.

51 Painful Spreading Cellulitis in an Injecting Drug User

Nicholas Kennedy

Case History

A 26-year-old man with a history of injecting drug use was admitted to hospital with a two-day history of pain and swelling of his left leg. He had no forearm veins left so he now injected into his femoral veins. His upper left thigh was red, swollen and very tender to touch. His temperature was 38.6°C, pulse rate 106 beats/min and blood pressure (BP) 105/66 mmHg. A clinical diagnosis of cellulitis was made. As he had no peripheral veins to cannulate, he was commenced on treatment with oral rather than intravenous flucloxacillin. On reviewing his condition two hours later, he had become confused, with worsening pain and spreading erythema of the thigh, a pulse rate of 120 beats/min, BP of 90/55 mmHg and poor urine output.

What was the most likely diagnosis at the time of admission and what would your differential diagnosis be?

Are you happy with his initial management? If not, how would you have managed him differently?

Should his antibiotic regimen be changed given the deterioration during his first two hours in hospital? If so, what would you change to?

Are any other therapeutic interventions required beyond changing his antimicrobial therapy?

Background

Skin and soft tissue infections (SSTIs) are very common in injecting drug users (IDUs). These infections can range from superficial ulcers and abscesses to life-threatening necrotizing infections with multisystem failure. Subcutaneous ('skin-popping') or intramuscular injection is a major risk factor for abscess formation and severe SSTI.

Groin injectors are at risk of cellulitis, abscess formation and bacteraemia (sometimes with associated endocarditis), along with coexistent ilio-femoral venous thromboses. Other vascular complications are also well recognized including pseudo-aneurysm. Imaging studies are therefore important for a full assessment.

Methicillin-susceptible *Staphylococcus aureus* (MSSA) and beta-haemolytic streptococci are the commonest organisms seen in IDUs with SSTI, although anaerobes and mixed flora are common if an abscess is present. More unusual organisms may also occur.

Recent Developments

Necrotizing soft tissue infection (NSTI) is a term that is used to describe a group of conditions that includes necrotizing cellulitis, necrotizing fasciitis (NF) and myonecrosis. Necrosis and thrombosis potentially involving skin, fat, fascia and muscle are central pathological processes for all of the NSTIs. IDUs are at significant risk from NSTI, with 80% of the cases of NSTI in a recent large, retrospective study in the USA occurring in IDUs (Frazee *et al.*, 2008).

A rise in invasive *Streptococcus pyogenes* infection has been seen in many countries since the 1980s. The spectrum of illness can range from mild cellulitis to life-threatening infections, including NF and streptococcal toxic shock syndrome (STSS). IDUs now account for 40% of severe *S. pyogenes* infections in young adults in the UK.

The 'textbook' features of NF (Table 51.1), the best-known NSTI, may occur late, if at all. Disproportionate pain and a rapidly progressive SSTI are therefore important clues. The underlying infection in NF can be monomicrobial, classically *S. pyogenes* in so-called type 2 NF, and may occur in conjunction with STSS. More commonly, NF is polymicrobial with a streptococcal, staphylococcal, Gram-negative or anaerobic infection present.

Table 51.1 Features of necrotizing fasciitis*

- Pain disproportionate to the physical findings
- Rapid progression despite antibiotic therapy
- Systemic toxicity
- Altered mental status
- Bullous lesions
- Cutaneous haemorrhage
- Skin anaesthesia
- Crepitus due to gas in the tissues

*These are the 'textbook' features. However, it is important to note that many of these features may be absent in the early stage of necrotizing fasciitis. Surgical exploration is the only way to reliably diagnose or exclude necrotizing fasciitis.

Severe NSTIs in IDUs due to spore-forming organisms, particularly various anaerobic *Clostridium* spp., are an important consideration (Table 51.2). Spores in contaminated heroin can survive the heating process prior to injecting. Oedema and myonecrosis are often prominent in clostridial NSTI. A dramatic outbreak occurred in Scotland in 2000 related to *C. novyi*, with skin- and muscle-popping identified as risk factors for severe infection. Injection-related tetanus and botulism (sometimes, but not invariably, associated with clinically obvious SSTI) are now also being seen (Table 51.2).

Methicillin-resistant *Staphylococcus aureus* (MRSA) is traditionally a healthcare-associated infection (HA-MRSA). However, the number of cases of community-acquired MRSA (CA-MRSA) infection has risen over the last decade, particularly in North America. IDUs are a known risk group for CA-MRSA in the USA, accounting for almost

Table 51.2 Soft tissue infections related to spore-forming bacteria in injecting drug users

Causative organism	Presentation
• *Clostridium novyi* • *Clostridium sordellii* • *Clostridium pefringens* • *Clostridium histolyticum* • *Bacillus cereus* • *Bacillus anthracis*	**Necrotizing soft tissue infections** Variable presentations which may include severe cellulitis, fasciitis, abscesses, myonecrosis, marked tissue oedema and cardiovascular collapse
• *Clostridium tetani*	**Tetanus** Neurotoxin initially results in muscular rigidity and local spasms at infection site, progressing to generalized tetanus
• *Clostridium botulinum*	**Botulism** Neurotoxin causes dysarthria, diplopia, dysphagia and a descending flaccid paralysis

half of such infections in California. In 2011 in the UK, CA-MRSA infections were still uncommon. Typically, UK strains are susceptible to clindamycin. Optimal antimicrobial therapy is unclear. In severe CA-MRSA SSTIs, parenteral therapy with a glycopeptide (vancomycin or teicoplanin), linezolid or daptomycin should be given, with combination therapy (e.g. linezolid, clindamycin and rifampicin) advised for cases where features of toxic shock or NF are present.

Antimicrobial management of severe SSTI and NSTI has to be guided to an extent by the clinical scenario and the suspected or isolated organisms. Combination therapy is needed. Staphylococcal (MSSA) infection must be adequately covered, for example with flucloxacillin. Importantly, clindamycin must be added if streptococcal NF is suspected, as it is efficacious during static growth phase, and may even inhibit toxin production. Gram-negative cover can be provided by gentamicin, a fluoroquinolone or a β-lactam/β-lactam inhibitor combination, whilst anaerobic cover is provided by clindamycin or metronidazole. Additional agents need to be considered if CA-MRSA is suspected.

Adjunctive treatment is vital in the management of severe SSTI or NSTI. This should include:

● Aggressive fluid resuscitation.
● Senior surgical review, as both the diagnosis and treatment of NF/NSTI require prompt surgical exploration and debridement – these are not conditions that can be reliably diagnosed clinically or treated with antibiotics alone.
● Critical care involvement with management in a high-dependency or intensive therapy unit and organ support if required.
● Consider intravenous immunoglobulin – severe *S. pyogenes* infection/STSS.
● Consideration of activated protein C, if criteria met.

Conclusion

● The differential diagnosis at admission in this case would include cellulitis, venous thrombosis, deep abscess or the early stages of a NSTI. The degree of swelling and tenderness should alert the clinician to the possibility of deep necrotizing SSTI.
● Several markers of sepsis were present on admission. Intravenous fluid resuscitation and parenteral antibiotic therapy, via a central line, was indicated.

● At two hours the patient fulfils the criteria for severe sepsis. Fluid resuscitation, critical care support, senior surgical review and a change to intravenous combination antibiotic therapy are urgently required. Intravenous clindamycin, flucloxacillin, benzylpenicillin and gentamicin would be suitable, unless there are strong reasons to suspect CA-MRSA. Urgent surgical exploration is the greatest priority.

Further Reading

Brett MM, Hood J, Brazier JS, Duerden BI, Hahné SJ. Soft tissue infections caused by spore-forming bacteria in injecting drug users in the United Kingdom. *Epidemiol Infect* 2005; **133**: 575–82.

Frazee BW, Fee C, Lynn J *et al.* Community-acquired necrotizing soft tissue infections: a review of 122 cases presenting to a single emergency department over 12 years. *J Emerg Med* 2008; **34**: 139–46.

Huang H, Flynn NM, King JH, Monchaud C, Morita M, Cohen SH. Comparisons of community-associated methicillin-resistant *Staphylococcus aureus* (MRSA) and hospital-associated MRSA infections in Sacramento, California. *J Clin Microbiol* 2006; **44**: 2423–7.

Lamagni TL, Neal S, Keshishian C *et al.* Severe *Streptococcus pyogenes* infections, United Kingdom, 2003–2004. *Emerg Infect Dis* 2008; **14**: 202–9.

Nathwani D, Morgan M, Masterton RG *et al.* Guidelines for UK practice for the diagnosis and management of methicillin-resistant *Staphylococcus aureus* (MRSA) infections presenting in the community. *J Antimicrob Chemother* 2008; **61**: 976–94.

Taylor A, Hutchinson S, Lingappa J *et al.* Severe illness and death among injecting drug users in Scotland: a case-control study. *Epidemiol Infect* 2005; **133**: 193–204.

PROBLEM

52 Anthrax in an Injecting Drug User

Erica Peters

Case History

A 42-year-old injecting drug user presented to the emergency department complaining of a painful groin. He felt generally unwell two days after injecting heroin into his femoral vein. Examination revealed a mildly tender groin with a small puncture wound. Striking oedema was present but there was minimal erythema. Blood pressure was normal. He appeared unwell and peripherally shut down. He had a sinus tachycardia of 120 beats/min but was afebrile with a normal respiratory rate. Baseline blood tests showed a C-reactive protein of 29 mg/l and normal white blood cell count and lactate. The patient was treated immediately with intravenous (IV) flucloxacillin and IV fluids. He became hypotensive after 12 hours and was taken to theatre as necrotizing fasciitis was considered likely. The wound was debrided and Gram stain of theatre tissue samples showed Gram-positive bacilli.

What is the differential diagnosis when the patient presents?

What is the likely microbiological diagnosis?

What is the classical presentation of this condition?

Background

Injecting drug users (IDUs) commonly present with skin and soft tissue infection. This is related to non-sterile injecting techniques, which facilitate the introduction of commensal skin and environmental flora into the tissues. The inguinal region, in particular, is often heavily contaminated with skin and faecal-type microbial flora. *Staphylococcus aureus* is the most common pathogen in these patients, probably due to a combination of poor hygiene and higher colonization rates of *S. aureus* among the injecting drug user population. Bacteraemia can occur from local lesions resulting in serious, deep-seated infections such as endocarditis and osteomyelitis. Blood-borne viral infections such as human immunodeficiency virus, hepatitis B and hepatitis C arise from sharing injecting equipment, and can be minimized through needle-exchange programmes and advice on sterile injecting techniques.

Acute soft tissue or bloodstream infection may also originate from contaminated drug or citric acid, which is often the medium used to dissolve the drug prior to injecting. Infection occurs following direct inoculation of vegetative organisms, such as staphylococci and streptococci, or spores, such as Clostridia, which can survive desiccation in the environment and contaminate the drug at source. Spores germinate under anaerobic conditions within the tissues and initiate secretion of pathogenic toxins. Clostridial species such as *Clostridium tetani*, *C. botulinum* and *C. novyi* are recognized in this context worldwide.

Another spore-forming pathogen, *Bacillus anthracis*, is found in many parts of the world, where there is potential for the contamination of opium products with animal manure during processing. This organism causes cutaneous anthrax, which is the most common form of anthrax infection and usually occurs as a zoonosis following direct skin inoculation. In endemic regions an eschar or black-centred ulcer with significant surrounding oedema is typical in those employed in high-risk occupations such as farmers or abattoir workers. Rarely bacteraemia can occur. Usually 7–10 days of oral antibiotics is sufficient for cutaneous disease. The far more serious inhalational anthrax is associated with people working with animal products (hides, wool, bone meal, etc.). Inhalational anthrax was also seen during the bioterrorist attacks in the USA in 2001. As the spores are small they can be aerosolized and subsequently inhaled to cause pneumonia. Gastrointestinal and central nervous system involvement are rare but well described. Mortality is high for systemic anthrax.

Management

In the case presented, the patient has a localized lesion with associated systemic symptoms. The differential diagnosis is cellulitis, groin abscess, venous thrombosis, compartment syndrome and necrotizing fasciitis. In contrast with necrotizing fasciitis, this patient had no severe localized pain or systemic sepsis at presentation. This concurs with a toxin-induced syndrome, which ultimately leads to rapid clinical deterioration and evolution of the systemic inflammatory response. Gram-positive staphylococci or streptococci are most frequently seen in skin and soft tissue infections in drug users, but in this case cultures demonstrated Gram-positive bacilli compatible with either *B. anthracis* or Clostridial species. Both can be readily identified using standard microbiological techniques but polymerase chain reaction and serology tests are also available for *B. anthracis*.

Given the signs of septic shock and significant localized oedema, *B. anthracis* was judged to be most likely. Local epidemiology is clearly important and in this case the infection had occurred in the context of a UK-wide outbreak of injecting drug use-related anthrax. The exotoxins secreted by *B. anthracis* are responsible for the cutaneous oedema which is frequently seen (Figure 52.1). Cardiovascular collapse, which can be refractory to fluid resuscitation and inotropes, and significant oozing and bleeding due to disseminated intravascular coagulation are also observed.

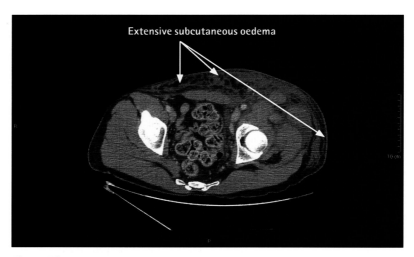

Figure 52.1 Abdominal computed tomography scan demonstrating gross abdominal wall oedema.

Urgent and repeated surgical debridement, systemic antibiotics and circulatory support are required. Expert advice should be sought from local infection specialists, with early involvement of public health personnel. The optimal antibiotic regimen and duration of therapy are not known, although inhalational anthrax requires at least 60 days of treatment as spores continue to germinate for weeks.

In most cases *B. anthracis* is susceptible to penicillin but there are some strains with inducible penicillinases which render the organism tolerant or resistant to first-line penicillins. The organism is naturally resistant to cephalosporins and co-trimoxazole.

Penicillin is not recommended as a sole agent until susceptibilities are known and ciprofloxacin or doxycycline might be more appropriate pending laboratory results. Clindamycin is known to suppress bacterial protein synthesis and subsequent release of toxins so may also be considered as an additional agent.

Recent Developments

Much research has been performed on the immunopathology of anthrax including a detailed understanding of toxin production, binding and effects. A specific anthrax antitoxin has been used in a few cases but there are no clinical trial data published evaluating its use. A preventative vaccine is available and is used in military settings or for those at high risk of exposure. Current work centres upon newer vaccines and vaccine delivery that could be produced and deployed for specific populations in the event of a widespread bioterrorism assault.

Conclusion

IDUs are at risk for a wide variety of infections. These usually involve common pathogens such as *S. aureus* and beta-haemolytic streptococci causing skin and soft tissue infections. The clinician should be alert to atypical presentations in IDUs, however, and consider a broad differential diagnosis including polymicrobial causes and toxin-producing pathogens. Anthrax may be rare in non-endemic zones but occasionally occurs in drug users, as well as representing a continued bioterrorism risk.

Further Reading

Centers for Disease Control and Prevention. Update: investigation of bioterrorism-related anthrax and interim guidelines for exposure management and antimicrobial therapy, October 2001. Available at: http://www.cdc.gov/mmwr/preview/mmwrhtml/mm5042a1.htm (accessed 12 08 11).

Cole C, Jones L, McVeigh J, Kicman A, Syed Q, Bellis M. Adulterants in illicit drugs: a review of empirical evidence. *Drug Test Anal* 2011; **3**: 89–96.

Gordon RJ, Lowy FD. Bacterial infections in drug users. *N Engl J Med* 2005; **353**: 1945–54.

Hahné SJ, White JM, Crowcroft NS *et al*. Tetanus in injecting drug users, United Kingdom. *Emerg Infect Dis* 2006; **12**: 709–10.

Swartz MN. Recognition and management of anthrax – an update. *N Engl J Med* 2001; **345**: 1621–6.

Ramsay CN, Stirling A, Smith J *et al*. An outbreak of infection with *Bacillus anthracis* in injecting drug users in Scotland. *Euro Surveill* 2010; **15** pii: 19465. Erratum in *Euro Surveill* 2010; **15** pii: 19469.

Stern EJ, Uhde KB, Shadomy SV, Messonnier N. Conference report on public health and clinical guidelines for anthrax. *Emerg Infect Dis* 2008; **14** pii: 07-0969.

Index